W9-DIG-820

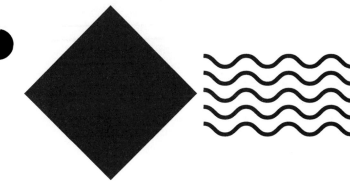

Student Learning Guide for

Basic Pharmacology for Nurses

Twelfth Edition

Bruce D. Clayton, BS, PharmD, RPh

Professor of Pharmacy Practice
College of Pharmacy & Health Sciences
Butler University
Indianapolis, Indiana

Yvonne N. Stock, RN, BSN, MS

Professor of Nursing
Health Occupations Department
Iowa Western Community College
Council Bluffs, Iowa

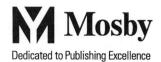

Mosby

Dedicated to Publishing Excellence

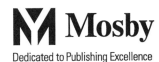

Mosby

Dedicated to Publishing Excellence

Student Learning Guide for Clayton and Stock
BASIC PHARMACOLOGY FOR NURSES (12/e)

Copyright © 2001, 1997 by Mosby, Inc.

All rights reserved. No part of this publication may be reproduced or transmitted in any form or by any means, electronic or mechanical, including photocopy, recording, or any information storage and retrieval system, without permission in writing from the publisher.

Permission to photocopy or reproduce solely for internal or personal use is permitted to libraries or other users registered with the Copyright Clearance Center, provided that the base fee of $4.00 per chapter plus $.10 per page is paid directly to the Copyright Clearance Center, 222 Rosewood Drive, Danvers, Massachusetts 01923. This consent does not extend to other kinds of copying, such as copying for general distribution, for advertising or promotional purposes, for creating new collected works, or for resale.

Although for mechanical reasons all pages of this publication are perforated, only those pages imprinted with a Mosby, Inc. copyright notice are intended for removal.

Mosby, Inc.
A Harcourt Health Sciences Company
11830 Westline Industrial Drive
St. Louis, Missouri 63146

Printed in the United States of America

International Standard Book Number 0-323-009778

00 01 02 03 04   /EB 9 8 7 6 5 4 3 2 1

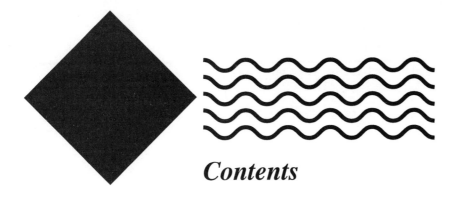

Contents

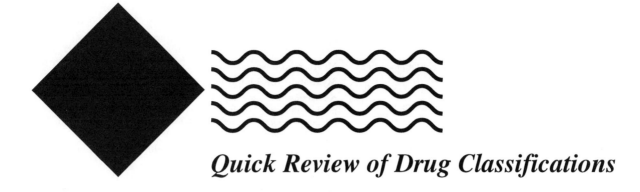

Quick Review of Drug Classifications

ACE inhibitors: These agents prevent the synthesis of angiotensin II, a potent vasoconstrictor; used to treat hypertension and heart failure.

Acetylcholinesterase inhibitors: These agents promote the accumulation of acetylcholine resulting in prolonged cholinergic effects.

Adrenergic: These drugs produce the effects similar to the neurotransmitter norepinephrine. Stimulation of $alpha_1$ receptors causes vasoconstriction of blood vessels; stimulation of $alpha_2$ receptors prevents further release of norepinephrine; stimulation of $beta_1$ receptors increases the heart rate; stimulation of $beta_2$ receptors causes bronchodilation, uterine relaxation, and vasodilation of peripheral blood vessels. When used for ophthalmology, these agents cause pupil dilation (mydriatic), increased outflow of aqueous humor, vasoconstriction, relaxation of ciliary muscle, and a decrease in the formation of aqueous humor.

Adrenergic blocking agents: These drugs inhibit the adrenergic system, thereby preventing stimulation of the adrenergic receptors.

Aminoglycosides: These drugs include gentamicin, tobramycin, and related antibiotics; noted for potentially dangerous toxicity.

Androgens: These drugs are steroid hormones that produce masculinizing effects.

Analgesics: (Narcotic and non-narcotic analgesics) These drugs relieve pain without producing loss of consciousness or reflex activity.

Anesthetics: These drugs cause a loss of sensation with or without a loss of consciousness (e.g., local anesthesia, general anesthesia).

Antacids: These drugs reduce the acidity of the gastric contents.

Antianginals: These drugs are used to prevent or treat attacks of angina pectoris.

Antianxiety: These drugs are used to treat anxiety symptoms or disorders. They are also known as minor tranquilizers or anxiolytics, although the term tranquilizer is generally avoided today to prevent the misperception that the patient is being tranquilized.

Antiarrhythmics: These drugs are used to correct cardiac arrhythmias. (An arrhythmia is any heart rate or rhythm other than normal sinus rhythm.)

Antibiotics: These agents are used to treat infections caused by pathogenic microbes; the term is often used interchangeably with antimicrobial agents.

Anticholinergic: These drugs, also known as cholinergic blocking agents, antispasmodics, or parasympatholytic agents, block the action of acetylcholine in the parasympathetic nervous system.

Anticoagulants: These drugs do not dissolve existing blood clots; they do prevent enlargement or extension of blood clots.

Anticonvulsants: These drugs suppress central nervous system abnormal neuronal activity and thereby prevent seizures.

Antidepressants: These drugs relieve depression

Antidiabetic: These drugs are also known as hypoglycemics. They include insulin, which is used to treat type 1 diabetes mellitus, and oral hypoglycemic agents, which are used in the treatment of type 2 diabetes mellitus.

Antidiarrheals: These agents relieve or control the symptoms of acute or chronic diarrhea.

Antiemetics: These drugs are used to prevent or treat nausea and vomiting.

Antifungals: These drugs are used to treat fungal infections.

Antiglaucoma: These drugs are used to reduce intraocular pressure found in glaucoma.

Antigout: These drugs are used in the treatment of active gout attacks or to prevent future episodes of gout.

Antihistamines: These drugs are used to treat allergy symptoms. They may also be used to treat motion sickness, insomnia, and other non-allergic reactions.

Antihypertensives: These agents are used to treat elevated blood pressure, hypertension.

Antilipemics: These drugs are used to reduce serum cholesterol and/or triglycerides.

Antimicrobials: These drugs are chemicals that eliminate living microorganisms pathogenic to the patient. They are also called antibiotics or anti-infectives.

Antineoplastics: These drugs are also called chemotherapy agents. They are used alone or in combination with other treatment modalities such as radiation, surgery, or biological response modifiers for the treatment of various types of cancer.

Antiparkinson's: These drugs are used in the treatment of Parkinson's disease and other dyskinesias.

Antiplatelets: These drugs prevent platelet clumping (aggregation) and thereby prevent an essential step in formation of a blood clot.

Antipsychotics: These drugs, also known as major tranquilizers or neuroleptics, are used in the treatment of severe mental illnesses. (The use of the word tranquilizer is being avoided today to prevent families from feeling the patient is tranquilized.)

Antipyretics: These drugs are used to reduce fevers associated with a variety of conditions.

Antispasmodics: These drugs are actually anticholinergic agents.

Antithyroid: These agents are used to treat the symptoms of hyperthyroidism. They are also known as thyroid hormone antagonists.

Antituberculins: These drugs are used to treat or prevent symptoms caused by *Mycobacterium tuberculosis*.

Antitussive: These drugs are used to suppress a cough by acting on the cough center of the brain.

Antiulcer agents: These drugs, such as histamine$_2$ antagonists, decrease the volume and increase the pH of gastric secretions.

Antivirals: These agents are used to treat infections caused by pathogenic viruses.

Bronchodilators: These drugs stimulate receptors within the tracheobronchial tree to relax and dilate the airway passages allowing for a greater volume of air to be exchanged thereby improving oxygenation.

Beta blockers: These agents inhibit the activity of sympathetic transmitters, norepinephrine, and epinephrine; used to treat angina, arrhythmias, hypertension, and glaucoma.

Calcium channel blockers: These drugs, also called calcium ion antagonists, slow channel blockers, or calcium ion influx inhibitors, inhibit the movement of calcium ions across the cell membrane. They are used to decrease arrhythmias, slow the rate of contraction of the heart, and cause vasodilation of blood vessels.

Carbonic anhydrase inhibitors: These drugs interfere with the production of aqueous humor and thereby reduce intraocular pressure associated with glaucoma.

Cell stimulating agents: These agents improve immune function by stimulating the activity of various immune cells.

Colony stimulating factors: These agents stimulate progenitor cells in bone marrow to increase numbers of leukocytes, thereby improving immune function.

Cholinergics: These drugs, also known as parasympathomimetics, produce effects that are similar to those of acetylcholine.

Cholinesterase inhibitors: These are enzymes that destroy acetylcholine, the cholinergic neurotransmitter.

Coating agents: This drug, sucralfate, forms a complex that adheres to the crater of an ulcer, protecting it from aggravation from gastric secretions.

Corticosteroids: These are hormones secreted by the adrenal cortex of the adrenal gland.

Cycloplegics: These drugs are anticholinergic agents that paralyze accommodation of the iris of the eye.

Cytotoxics: These are agents that cause direct cell death; often used for cancer chemotherapy.

Decongestants: These drugs act by reducing swelling in the nasal passages caused by a common cold or allergic rhinitis.

Digestants: These are combination products used to treat various digestive disorders and to supplement deficiencies of natural digestive enzymes.

Digitalis glycosides: These drugs increase the force of contraction and slow the heart rate, thereby improving cardiac output.

Diuretics: These are drugs that act to increase the flow of urine.

Emetics: Drugs used to induce vomiting.

Estrogens: Steroids that cause feminizing effects.

Expectorants: These drugs liquefy mucous by stimulating the natural lubricant fluids from the bronchial glands.

Fluoroquinolones These drugs include ciprofloxacin and related agents; widely used broad-spectrum antibiotics.

Gastric stimulants: These drugs are used to increase stomach contractions, relax the pyloric valve, and increase peristalsis in the gastrointestinal tract, resulting in an increase in gastric transit time and emptying of the intestinal tract.

Glucocorticoids: These drugs are also known as adrenocorticosteroids and are used to regulate carbohydrate, fat, and protein metabolism.

Gonadal hormones: These are hormones produced by the testis in the male and ovaries in the female.

Herbals: These are plant products usually sold as food supplements; may have pharmacologic effects that are not evaluated or regulated by the FDA

Histamine H$_2$ Antagonists: These drugs decrease the volume and increase the pH of gastric secretions during both the day and the night.

Hyperuricemics: These drugs are used to decrease the production of and increase the excretion of uric acid.

Hypnotics: These are drugs used to produce sleep.

Insulins: Insulin is a hormone required for glucose transport to the cells.

Lactation suppressants: These drugs are used to prevent physiologic lactation.

Laxatives: These drugs act by a variety of mechanisms to treat constipation.

Low molecular weight heparins: These drugs are anticoagulants used for the prophylactic treatment of pulmonary thromboembolism and deep vein thrombosis.

Macrolides: These drugs include erythromycin, azithromycin, and related antibiotics.

MAO inhibitors: These agents block monoamine oxidase, thereby preventing the degradation of norepinephrine and serotonin.

Mineralocorticoids: Steroids that cause the kidneys to retain sodium and water.

Miotics: These drugs cause constriction of the iris.

Mucolytics: These drugs reduce the thickness and stickiness of pulmonary secretions by acting directly on the mucous plugs to dissolve them.

Muscle relaxants: These drugs relieve muscle spasms.

Mydriatics: These drugs cause dilation of the iris.

Neuromuscular blockers: These are skeletal muscle relaxants used to produce muscle relaxation during anesthesia to reduce the use and side effects of general anesthetics, used to ease endotracheal intubation and prevent laryngospasm.

Nitrates: These are agents that degrade to nitric oxide, a potent vasodilator used to treat angina.

Nonsteroidal anti-inflammatory drugs (NSAIDs): These drugs, known as NSAIDS or "aspirin-like" drugs, are chemically unrelated to the salicylates but are prostaglandin inhibitors.

Opioids: These centrally acting analgesic agents are related to morphine.

Oral contraceptives: These drugs are used for birth control.

Oral hypoglycemics: These agents are used in type 2 diabetes mellitus to improve glucose metabolism and lower blood glucose levels.

Progestins: These steroids regulate endometrial and myometrial function; used alone or in combination with estrogen for oral contraception.

Protease inhibitors: Saquinavir, ritonavir, indinavir, and related drugs that block the maturation of human immunodeficiency viruses; used for HIV infections.

Salicylates: These drugs are effective as analgesics, antipyretics and antiinflammatory agents.

Sedatives: These drugs are given to produce relaxation and rest, but do not necessarily produce sleep.

Selective serotonin reuptake inhibitors (SSRIs): Antidepressants that act by specifically blocking the reuptake of serotonin.

Serotonin Antagonists: These agents block serotonin; used to prevent emesis induced by chemotherapy, radiation therapy, and surgery.

Statins (HMG-CoA reductase inhibitors): Agents that block the synthesis of cholesterol

Stool softeners or fecal softeners: These drugs draw water into the stool, thereby softening it.

Sympatholytics: These drugs interfere with the storage and release of norepinephrine.

Sympothomimetics: These agents mimic the action of dopamine, norepinephrine, and epinephrine.

Thyroid hormone antagonists: These drugs are used to counteract /block the action of excessive formation of thyroid hormones.

Thyroid hormones: These drugs are used to replace thyroid hormones that are not being produced or are not produces in sufficient quantities to meet the body's physiologic needs.

Thrombolytics: These drugs include, alteplase, anistreplase, streptokinase or urokinase; given to dissolve existing blood clots.

Tricyclic Antidepressants: These antidepressants, such as doxepin, amitriptyline, imipramine, inhibit the reuptake of norepinephrine and serotonin

Uricosuric agents: These drugs act on the tubules of the kidneys to enhance the excretion of uric acid.

Urinary analgesics: These agents produce a local anesthetic effect on the mucosa of the ureters and bladder to relieve burning, pain, urgency, and frequency associated with urinary tract infections (UTIs).

Urinary antimicrobials: These drugs are substances that are excreted and concentrated in the urine in sufficient amounts to have an antiseptic effect on the urine and the urinary tract.

Uterine stimulants: These drugs increase the frequency or strength of uterine contractions.

Uterine relaxants: These drugs are used to primarily prevent preterm labor and delivery.

Vaccines: These are suspensions of live, attenuated, or killed bacteria or viruses.

Vasodilators: These agents relax the arteriolar smooth muscle.

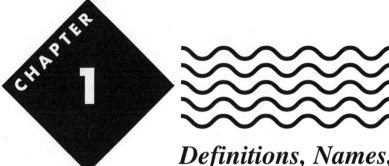

Syllabus

Definitions, Names, Standards, and Informational Sources

CHAPTER CONTENT

CHAPTER OBJECTIVES

Definitions

1. State the origin and definition of *pharmacology*.
2. Explain the meaning of *therapeutic methods*.

Drug Names (USA)

1. Describe the process used to name drugs.
2. Differentiate among the *chemical, generic, official,* and *brand* names of medicines.

Drug Names (Canada)

1. Differentiate between the *official* and *proper* names of medicines.

Sources of Drug Standards (USA)

1. List official sources of drug standards.

Sources of Drug Standards (Canada)

1. List official sources of drug standards.

Sources of Drug Information (USA)

1. List and describe literature resources for researching prescription and nonprescription medications.
2. List and describe literature resources for researching drug interactions and drug compatibilities.

Sources of Drug Information (Canada)

1. Describe the organization of the *Compendium of Pharmaceuticals and Specialties* and the information contained in each colored section.
2. Describe the organization of *Nonprescription Drug Reference for Health Professionals*.
3. Describe the organization of *Compendium of Nonprescription Drugs*.

Sources of Patient Information

1. Cite literature resources for reviewing information to be given to the patient concerning prescribed medications.

Drug Legislation (USA)

1. List legislative acts controlling drug use and abuse.
2. Differentiate among Schedule I, II, III, IV, and V medications, and describe nursing responsibilities associated with the administration of each type of drug.

Drug Legislation (Canada)

1. List legislative acts controlling drug use and abuse.
2. Differentiate between Schedule F and G medications, and describe nursing responsibilities with each.

New Drug Development

1. Describe the procedure outlined by the FDA to develop and market new medicines.

KEY WORDS

pharmacology
therapeutic methods
medicine
drug
chemical name
generic name
official name
trademark
brand name
proprietary name
drug classifications

over-the-counter (OTC) drugs
illegal drugs
United States Pharmacopeia/ National Formulary (USP/NF)
British Pharmacopoeia
Pharmacopee Francaise
American Drug Index
American Hospital Formulary Service

Copyright © 2001 by Mosby, Inc. All rights reserved.

Drug Interaction Facts
Drug Facts and
    Comparisons
Handbook on Injectable
    Drugs
Handbook of
    Nonprescription
    Drugs
Martindale—The
    Complete Drug
    Reference
Medical Letter
Physicians' Desk
    Reference (PDR)
Mosby's GenRx
Electronic Databases
Compendium of
    Pharmaceutical and
    Specialties (CPS)
Nonprescription Drug
    Reference for Health
    Professionals
Compendium of
    Nonprescription
    Drugs

United States
    Pharmacopeia
    Dispensing
    Information (USP DI)
Tyler's Honest Herbal
Federal Food, Drug, and
    Cosmetic Act
Controlled Substances Act
Scheduled Drugs
Food and Drugs Act, 1927
Food and Drug
    Regulations 1953,
    1954, 1979
Nonprescription drugs
Preclinical Research
Clinical Research
New Drug Application
    Review
Postmarketing
    Surveillance
Health Orphans

ASSIGNMENTS

Read textbook pages 2 to 13.
Study Review Sheets for Chapter 1.
Study the Key Words associated with the chapter content.
Complete Chapter 1 Practice Quiz.
Complete Chapter 1 Exam.

COLLABORATIVE ACTIVITIES

Complete the following activities and questions to prepare for in-class discussion and group work that may be assigned by the instructor.

A. Controlled Substances

Turn to p. 79 and examine the names of the medicines listed on the controlled substance inventory form. Compare the drugs listed with those found on the controlled substance inventory form at your clinical practice setting assignment. What additional drugs are listed in the clinical practice setting? Discuss possible reasons for such differences.

B. New Drugs/Research

Discuss the nurse's role in clinical research involving new drug products being administered in a clinical site.

C. Activity Designed to Acquaint the Student with the *PDR*

Section 2 of the *PDR*: Identify the generic and brand names of the following drugs using this section of the *PDR*:

Generic name: *Brand name:*

1. Theophylline ethylenediamine extended release tablets
2. Indomethacin suppositories
3. Rifampin tablets

Section 3 of the *PDR*: Give an example of a drug in the following therapeutic classes:

1. Hypolipidemic agent—
2. Proton pump inhibitor—
3. Calcium channel blocker—

Section 4 of *PDR*: A patient describes a medicine she is taking at home as about 3/4" long, capsule-shaped, with oval ends, orange with MSD697 printed on one side. Using this information, can you identify the medication using Section 4? If unable to identify it, what would you do?

Section 5 of *PDR*: Examine and list the major categories of information found in a package insert that accompanies a drug.

Discuss the value of information found in a package insert to the nurse in the clinical setting.

D. Electronic Database Activity

Go to the library in your school and have the librarian demonstrate the electronic database services available for the study of pharmacology.

Copyright © 2001 by Mosby, Inc. All rights reserved.

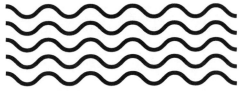

Practice Quiz

Definitions, Names, Standards, and Informational Sources

Complete the following statements or answer questions using key words from Chapter 1.

1. The study of drugs and the actions they have in the human body is _____.
2. The actual substance that causes the response in the living organism is a/an _____ .
3. How do chemical names differ from brand names and generic names?

Use the textbook and other drug resources (e.g., PDR) to identify the brand name or generic name and additional brand names for each drug listed.

Generic name:	Brandname:	Other Brandnames:
4. Aspirin		
5.	Tylenol®	
6.	Pepto-Bismol®	
7.	Maalox®	
8. Ibuprofen		
9.	Tums®	

Summarize the content found in each of the following pharmacy resource books:

10. *American Drug Index*

11. *American Hospital Formulary Service, Drug Information*

12. *Facts and Comparisons*

13. *Martindale—The Complete Drug Reference*

14. *Handbook of Nonprescription Drugs*

15. *Medical Letter*

16. *Physicians' Desk Reference* (PDR)

CONTROLLED SUBSTANCES

For each medicine listed, identify the DEA schedule. Use the textbook and other resources.

Medicine	DEA Schedule
17. Darvocet N®	C-
18. Diazepam	C-
19. Flurazepam	C-
20. LevoDromoran	C-
21. Meperidine	C-
22. Morphine Sulfate	C-
23. Tylenol® with codeine no. 2	C-
24. Tylenol® with codeine no. 3	C-
25. Tylenol® with codeine no. 4	C-
26. Percodan®	C-
27. Tylox® Capsules	C-

DRUG LEGISLATION

Essay

28. What is the purpose of the Controlled Substances Act of 1970?
29. When can a nurse be in possession of controlled substances without it being considered a crime?
30. What information is found in *Tyler's Honest Herbal* reference and of what significance is it to the nurse during patient education?
31. What drug information resources are immediately available on the clinical unit where you are assigned? Is there an electronic database available in addition to hardcopy materials?

Copyright © 2001 by Mosby, Inc.   All rights reserved.

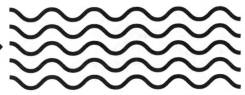

Syllabus

Principles of Drug Action and Drug Interactions

CHAPTER CONTENT

Basic principles (p. 14)
Drug action (p. 17)
Variable factors influencing drug action (p. 17)
Drug interactions (p. 18)

CHAPTER OBJECTIVES

Basic Principles

1. Identify five basic principles of drug action.
2. Explain nursing assessments necessary to evaluate potential problems associated with the absorption of medications.
3. Describe nursing interventions that can enhance drug absorption.
4. List three categories of drug administration and state the routes of administration for each category.
5. Differentiate between general and selective drug distribution mechanisms.
6. Name the process that inactivates drugs.
7. Identify the meaning and significance to the nurse of the term *half-life* when used in relation to drug therapy.

Drug Action

1. Compare and contrast the following terms used with regard to medications: *desired action, side effects, adverse effects, allergic reactions, and idiosyncratic reactions.*

Variable Factors Influencing Drug Action

1. List factors that cause variations in absorption, metabolism, distribution, and excretion of drugs.

Drug Interactions

1. State the mechanism by which drug interactions may occur.
2. Differentiate among the following terms used with regard to medications: *additive effect, synergistic effect, antagonistic effect, displacement, interference, and incompatibility.*

KEY WORDS

receptors
agonists
antagonists
partial agonists
ADME
pharmacokinetics
absorption
enteral
parenteral
percutaneous
distribution
drug blood level
metabolism
biotransformation
excretion
half-life
desired action
side effects
adverse effects

toxicity
idiosyncratic reaction
allergic reaction
urticaria
hives
carcinogenicity
teratogen
placebo
tolerance
drug dependence
drug accumulation
drug interaction
antagonistic effect
unbound drug
displacement
additive effect
interference
synergistic effect
incompatibility

ASSIGNMENTS

Read textbook, pp. 14-20.
Study key words associated with chapter content.
Complete Review Study Sheets for Chapter 2.
Complete Chapter 2 Practice Quiz.
Complete Chapter 2 Exam.

Copyright © 2001 by Mosby, Inc.   All rights reserved.

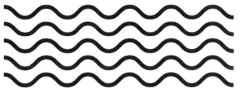

Review Sheet

Principles of Drug Action and Drug Interactions

Note to the student: Understanding the vocabulary associated with the study of pharmacology is fundamental to understanding the remaining information presented in the textbook. Therefore, the first step is to define and memorize the vocabulary. The second step is to apply the vocabulary learned during the pharmacology course. The third step in learning pharmacology is to apply the vocabulary during the actual clinical practice of nursing.

The QUESTION column and the ANSWER column have been offset so you can cover the answer while reading the question, allowing you to assess your knowledge. Define the following vocabulary.

Question	**Answer**
1. Receptors	
2. Agonists	1. Sites on the cells where chemical bonding of drugs occurs are receptors.
3. Antagonists	2. Drugs that stimulate a response at a receptor site are agonists.
4. Partial agonists	3. Drugs that attach to receptor sites, but do NOT stimulate a response are antagonists.
5. ADME	4. Drugs that interact with a receptor to stimulate a response and concurrently inhibit other responses are partial agonists.
6. Pharmacokinetics	5. ADME is an abbreviation for the four stages of drug processing: absorption, distribution, metabolism, and excretion.
	6. Pharmacokinetics is the study of the mathematical relationship between the absorption, distribution, metabolism, and excretion of medicines.
7. Absorption	7. Absorption is the process by which a drug is made available to the body fluids for distribution.
8. Enteral	8. The enteral route of drug administration is placed directly into the gastrointestinal tract by oral, rectal, or nasogastric routes.
9. Parenteral	9. Parenteral routes of drug administration are subcutaneous (SC), intramuscular (IM), or intravenous (IV) injection.
10. Percutaneous	10. Percutaneous drug administration is done via inhalation, sublingual, or topical administration.
11. Distribution	11. The term distribution refers to the ways in which drugs are transported by the circulating body fluids to the sites of action (receptors) for metabolism and excretion.
12. Drug blood level	

Copyright © 2001 by Mosby, Inc. All rights reserved.

13. Biotransformation (Metabolism)

14. Excretion

15. Half-life

16. Desired action

17. Side effects

18. Adverse effects

19. Idiosyncratic reaction

20. Allergic reactions

21. Urticaria (hives)

22. Carcinogenicity

23. Teratogen

24. Placebo
25. Tolerance

26. Drug dependence

27. Drug accumulation

28. Drug interaction

12. The drug blood level measures the amount of a drug present in the blood to determine if it is within the therapeutic range, below the range (subtherapeutic), or above the range (toxic).

13. The process by which a drug is inactivated (broken down). The terms *metabolism* and *biotransformation* are used interchangeably.

14. Excretion of a drug is the elimination of the active drug or its metabolites from the body.

15. The time required for one-half, or 50%, of the drug administered to be excreted from the body.

16. The achievement of the expected response to the drug administered.

17. Most side effects are predictable responses seen when a specific drug is administered. (The drug monographs throughout the textbook will give suggested nursing actions that can make these anticipated reactions more tolerable to the patient.)

18. Adverse effects are side effects that are more serious and require reporting to the physician for further orders on how to manage these reactions.
These are sometimes referred to as "drug toxicity" reactions. Adverse effects are labeled "side effects to report" throughout this textbook.

19. Idiosyncratic reactions are reactions that are not predictable; they are unusual or abnormal responses to the drug administered.

20. An allergic reaction, also called a *hypersensitivity reaction*, occurs in an individual who has previously taken the drug and been sensitized to it. With repeat administration, antibodies formed when the drug was first given respond to the repeated exposure producing an undesirable response, such as severe itching, urticaria (hives), or in more severe cases, collapse of the respiratory and cardiovascular systems, known as *anaphylactic reaction* or *anaphylaxis*, a life-threatening situation.

21. Urticaria or hives is an elevated irregular patch-like rash on the skin accompanied by itching.

22. Carcinogenicity is the ability of a drug to cause living cells to be altered (mutate) and become cancerous.

23. A drug that causes birth defects is a teratogen.

24. A placebo is a drug dosage form that contains no active ingredients.

25. Tolerance occurs when higher doses of a drug are required to achieve the same effects that a lower dose once achieved.

26. Drug dependence, also called *addiction* or *habituation*, occurs when the individual is no longer able to control the ingestion of the drug.

27. Drug accumulation occurs when there is an excess amount of a drug in the body due to a number of possible physiologic variables. This can result in drug toxicity.

Copyright © 2001 by Mosby, Inc. All rights reserved.

29. Unbound drug

30. Additive effect

31. Synergistic effect

32. Antagonistic effect

33. Displacement

34. Interference

35. Incompatibility

28. Drug interaction occurs when one drug being administered changes the action of other the drugs being used at the same time.
29. Unbound or free drug is the active amount of drug available to achieve the desired physiologic response of the drug.
30. Additive effect occurs when two drugs with similar actions have an increased effect.
31. Synergistic effect occurs when the combined effect of two drugs is greater than the sum of the effect of each drug given alone.
32. Antagonistic effect occurs when one drug interferes with the action of another.
33. Displacement occurs when one drug is moved from the protein binding sites by a second drug. This usually increases the activity of the first drug because it is now unbound.
34. Interference occurs when one drug inhibits the metabolism or excretion of a second drug, causing increased activity of the second drug.
35. Incompatibility occurs when one drug is chemically incompatible with another drug, resulting in deterioration of the drug.

Copyright © 2001 by Mosby, Inc. All rights reserved.

CHAPTER 2

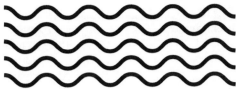

Practice Quiz

Principles of Drug Action and Drug Interactions

TRUE OR FALSE

DIRECTIONS: Mark "T" for true or "F" for false for each statement. <u>Correct all false statements.</u>

_____ 1. "Percutaneous route" is the administration of drugs by subcutaneous, intramuscular, or intravenous injection.

_____ 2. Enteral route is the administration of drugs to the gastrointestinal tract.

_____ 3. Agonists stimulate a response at a receptor site on the cells.

_____ 4. Partial agonists stimulate some responses, while inhibiting others, at a receptor site on the cells.

_____ 5. Parenteral route is the administration of drugs by inhalation, sublingual, or topical methods.

_____ 6. Receptors are specific sites within the body where a drug acts.

_____ 7. Antagonists cause a drug response at a receptor site.

_____ 8. Absorption refers to the ability of a drug to be integrated into the body fluids.

_____ 9. Metabolism is the activation of a drug for use by the body.

_____ 10. Distribution is the transportation of a drug within the body fluids for utilization within the body.

_____ 11. Excretion of a drug is the elimination of a drug from the body.

_____ 12. Biotransformation is another term for excretion of a drug.

_____ 13. Drug blood level is a measurement of the amount of drug present in the blood at the specific time of the blood draw.

COMPLETION

Finish each of the following statements using the correct term.

14. A drug interaction that produces an increased action is known as a(n) _____ interaction.

15. Two drugs with similar actions that produce an effect substantially greater than either drug administered alone is _____.

16. When one drug moves the original drug administered from a binding site to produce an increased drug effect, this is known as _____.

17. Drug _____ is defined as one drug chemically destroying a second drug if mixed together prior to administration.

18. Drug tolerance is _____.

19. Drug dependence is _____.

MULTIPLE CHOICE

Choose the BEST answer from those provided.

_____ 20. The primary routes for drug excretion are
   a. skin and lungs.
   b. gastrointestinal tract and the skin.
   c. renal tubules and GI tract.
   d. lungs and renal tubules.

_____ 21. Drug distribution occurs by
   a. decreasing body protein levels.
   b. transport in blood and lymphatic systems.
   c. keeping drug at toxic levels.
   d. increasing the amount of adipose tissue.

_____ 22. A partial agonist is a drug that stimulates
   a. action at receptor sites within the circulating blood.
   b. one response and inhibits another response.
   c. no response when attached to a receptor site.
   d. a response at a receptor site.

_____ 23. Another name for an idiosyncratic reaction is a(n)
   a. allergic reaction.
   b. toxic reaction.
   c. teratogenic reaction.
   d. drug over-response.

Copyright © 2001 by Mosby, Inc. All rights reserved.

_____ 24. The literature states that the half-life of a particular drug is eight hours. This means _____% of the drug will have been excreted in this time period.
   a. 25
   b. 30
   c. 50
   d. 75

_____ 25. A *desired* drug action is
   a. the predictable/usual response to the drug.
   b. an unusual or idiosyncratic response to a drug.
   c. capable of inducing cell mutations.
   d. the development of symptoms that should be reported to the prescribing physician.

Copyright © 2001 by Mosby, Inc.   All rights reserved.

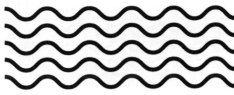

CHAPTER 3

Syllabus

Drug Action Across the Life Span

CHAPTER CONTENT

Changing Drug Action Across the Life Span (p. 20)
    Drug Absorption (p. 21)
    Drug Distribution (p. 21)
    Drug Metabolism (p. 22)
    Drug Elimination (p. 22)
Monitoring Drug Therapy (p. 23)

CHAPTER OBJECTIVES

1. Discuss the effects of age on drug action.
2. Cite major factors associated with drug absorption, distribution, metabolism, and excretion in the younger and the older populations.
3. Cite major factors associated with drug absorption, distribution, metabolism, and excretion in men and women.

KEY WORDS

passive diffusion
hydrolysis
intestinal transit
protein binding
drug metabolism
metabolites
polypharmacy

ASSIGNMENTS

Read textbook, pp. 20-23.
Study Review Sheet for Chapter 3.
Study Key Words associated with chapter content.
Complete Chapter 3 Practice Quiz.
Complete Chapter 3 Exam.

Copyright © 2001 by Mosby, Inc.   All rights reserved.

Review Sheet

Drug Action Across the Life Span

The QUESTION column and the ANSWER column have been offset so that you can cover the answer while reading the question, allowing you to assess your knowledge.

Question	Answer
1. What are common terms used to refer to individuals of different ages up to five years old?	
2. What is the underlying rationale for the erratic absorption of intramuscular (IM) drugs in both the neonate and the geriatric population?	1. <38 weeks = premature, 0-1 months = newborn or neonate, 1-24 months = infant or baby, 1-5 years = young child.
3. Define *passive diffusion*. (Research other sources.)	2. Differences in muscle mass and blood flow to muscles, and muscular inactivity in the bedridden patient.
4. Define *carrier-mediated diffusion*. (Research other sources.)	3. Passive diffusion is the most common mechanism associated with drug absorption. It requires no cellular energy and involves the movement of a drug from an area of high concentration to an area of low concentration.
5. Define *active transport*. (Research other sources.)	4. Carrier-mediated diffusion, or facilitated transport or diffusion, occurs when the drug molecules combine with a carrier substance such as an enzyme or other protein. An example is glucose combining with insulin to be carried from the bloodstream into the cell, moving from an area of high concentration (the bloodstream) to an area of low concentration (the cell). In other words, the drug needs help to pass across the cell membrane and the insulin passively provides the transport. This passive process requires no cellular energy.
6. State two factors that influence drug absorption from the gastrointestinal tract.	5. Active transport involves the movement of drug molecules from an area of low concentration to an area of high concentration. This process requires cellular energy to accomplish the movement.
7. Summarize the gastric pH in a premature infant, newborn, infant, adult, and elder.	6. Passive diffusion and gastric emptying time influence the absorption of drugs in the intestinal tract. Both passive diffusion and gastric emptying time are dependent on pH.

Copyright © 2001 by Mosby, Inc. All rights reserved.

8. Compare gastric emptying time in a premature infant, adult, and elder.

7. The gastric pH values are:
   premature   6-8
   newborn   6-8; decreases to 2-4 in 24 hours
   infant   1-3
   adult   1-3
   elder   pH is increased due to decreasing number of acid-secreting cells

9. Look up the term *hydrolysis* in a dictionary.

8. Premature infants and geriatric patients have slower gastric emptying time; therefore, the drug is in contact with the absorptive tissue longer. This may result in more absorption and a higher serum concentration of the drug in the blood.

10. In the newborn, what factor affects the absorption of drugs during the process of hydrolysis?
11. If gastric emptying time increases, what happens to the speed of absorption of a drug?

9. Hydrolysis is the chemical alteration or decomposition of a compound with water.
10. In an infant, the absence of enzymes needed for hydrolysis of certain drugs influences the ability of the drug to be absorbed.
11. The faster the gastric emptying time, the less time the drug has to be absorbed; therefore, drug absorption is decreased.

12. What effect does the route of drug administration have on drug absorption?

13. Why is transdermal absorption of a drug in an elder difficult to predict?

12. In general, drug absorption is affected by: drug dosage form (e.g., liquid verses enteric-coated tablets); route of drug administration (e.g., oral, intramuscular, inhalation, etc.); solubility of the drug; gastrointestinal function; the condition of the absorptive surface (e.g., inflamed, open skin area verses intact skin); and blood flow to and from the site.

14. What factors affect drug distribution?

13. In an elder, there is decreased dermal thickness that may increase drug absorption; however, there may be drying and wrinkling and decreased hair follicles that decrease absorption. There is often decreased cardiac output, which results in decreased blood flow to the tissues (decreased tissue perfusion), which results in decreased drug absorption.

14. Distribution is dependent on pH, body water concentration (intracellular, extracellular, and total body water), presence and quantity of fat tissue, protein binding, cardiac output, and regional blood flow.

15. Examine Table 3-1 on p. 22 of the text. Compare the total percent of body water in a premature infant, a full-term infant, a 1 year old, and a male adult. What conclusion(s) did you reach?

15. The younger the individual, the higher the percent of the total body water.

16. What effect will a higher percent of total body water have on drug absorption?

16. A higher percent of total body water means drugs that are water soluble will be more rapidly distributed and the individual may require a higher dose of these drugs. Conversely, fat-soluble drugs would be poorly absorbed.

17. Research the meaning of lipid-soluble and water-soluble.

17. Water-soluble drugs have an affinity for body fluids and are quickly absorbed and excreted through the kidneys; therefore, water-soluble drugs often have a shorter half-life. Lipid-soluble drugs have an affinity for fat tissue in the body and will often have a longer half-life.

18. Define *protein binding*.

Copyright © 2001 by Mosby, Inc.   All rights reserved.

19. What happens to the concentration of albumin in the body after the age 40?

20. What happens to the rate of drug metabolism in the elderly?

21. How functional is the renal filtration system of preterm infants and of full-term newborns when compared to that of an adult?

22. What effect do age and renal function have on drug dosages?

23. What test is used as the best predictor to estimate renal function in the elderly?

24. Define *polypharmacy*.

18. Protein binding occurs when a drug binds to proteins in the body, such as albumin. When "bound," the drug is not "free" or actively available for use at the receptor sites for action.

19. Total albumin concentration decreases after age 40, while other proteins increase. This results in an increase in unbound drug making more free drug available for action and metabolism.

20. The number of functioning hepatic cells and the blood flow decreases with aging, resulting in slower drug metabolism. As drug metabolism decreases, drug doses must be reduced to prevent accumulation of the drug, producing toxicity.

21. At birth, preterm infants have approximately 15% and full-term infants have approximately 35% of the renal capacity of an adult.

22. Drug doses must be adjusted so an adequate, therapeutic serum blood concentration is maintained. Increased age and decreased renal function often require a reduced dosage.

23. The urine creatinine test is used to estimate renal function in the elderly.

24. Polypharmacy is the use of multiple drugs concurrently.

Copyright © 2001 by Mosby, Inc. All rights reserved.

Practice Quiz

Drug Action Across the Life Span

TRUE OR FALSE

Directions: Mark "T" for true and "F" for false for each statement. <u>Correct all false statements.</u>

_____ 1. The elderly population includes persons 65 years and older.

_____ 2. Absorption of drugs administered intramuscularly is consistent and predictable.

_____ 3. Transdermal drug absorption has a predictable rate.

_____ 4. Enteric-coated and sustained-release tablets are absorbed erratically if crushed.

_____ 5. Passive diffusion requires cellular energy.

_____ 6. The gastric emptying time of the elder and the premature infant are slow and result in increased drug absorption.

_____ 7. Hydrolysis involves the chemical breakdown of a compound, such as a drug, in water.

_____ 8. The elderly patient has a greater percentage of total body fluid than an infant.

_____ 9. Drug elimination is affected by the number of functional renal tubules.

_____ 10. Albumin is a protein to which drugs bind for transport.

_____ 11. "Unbound" drug is the active portion of the drug dose available for the desired drug action.

_____ 12. "Bound" drug is the portion of the drug causing the desired drug action.

_____ 13. The term "infant" is used to signify babies 0-1 month of age.

Copyright © 2001 by Mosby, Inc.   All rights reserved.

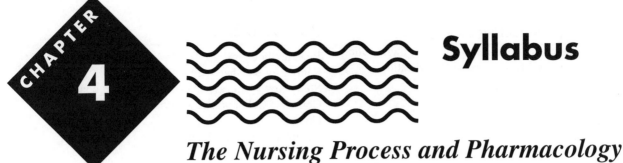

CHAPTER 4

Syllabus

The Nursing Process and Pharmacology

CHAPTER CONTENT

The Nursing Process (p. 23)
Relating the Nursing Process to Pharmacology (p. 32)

CHAPTER OBJECTIVES

The Nursing Process

1. Identify the purpose for using the nursing process methodology.
2. State the five steps in the nursing process and describe in terms of a problem-solving method used in nursing practice.

Assessment

1. Describe the components of the assessment process.
2. Compare current methods used to collect, organize, and analyze information about the health care needs of patients and their significant others.

Nursing Diagnosis

1. Define *nursing diagnosis* and discuss the wording used in formulating nursing diagnosis statements.
2. Define *collaborative problem.*
3. Differentiate between a nursing diagnosis and a medical diagnosis.
4. Differentiate between problems that require formulation of nursing diagnoses and those categorized as collaborative problems, which may not require nursing diagnosis statements.

Planning

1. Identify the steps included in the planning of nursing care.
2. Explain the process of prioritizing individual patient needs utilizing Maslow's hierarchy of needs.
3. Formulate measurable goal statements for a patient for whom you are actively caring in the clinical practice setting.
4. State the behavioral responses around which goal statements revolve when planning a patient's discharge.
5. Identify the purposes of a patient care plan.

6. Differentiate between nursing interventions and therapeutic outcomes.

Nursing Intervention or Implementation

1. Compare the types of nursing functions classified as dependent, interdependent, and independent, and give examples of each.

Evaluating and Recording Therapeutic Outcomes

1. Describe the evaluatory process used to establish whether patient behaviors are consistent with the identified short-term, intermediate, or long-term goals.

Relating the Nursing Process to Pharmacology

Assessment

1. State the information that should be obtained as a part of the medication history.
2. Identify primary, secondary, and tertiary sources of information used to build a patient information base.

Nursing Diagnosis

1. Define *problem.*
2. Describe the process used to identify factors that could result in patient problems when medications are prescribed.
3. Review several drug monographs to identify information that may result in patient problems from the medication therapy.

Planning

1. Identify steps used to plan nursing care in relation to a medication regimen prescribed for a patient.
2. Describe an acceptable method of organizing, implementing, and evaluating the patient education delivered.
3. Practice developing short-term and long-term patient education objectives and have them critiqued by the instructor.

Nursing Intervention or Implementation

1. Differentiate among dependent, interdependent, and independent nursing actions and give an example of each.

Copyright © 2001 by Mosby, Inc. All rights reserved.

Evaluating Therapeutic Outcomes

1. Describe the procedure for evaluating the therapeutic outcomes obtained from prescribed medication therapy.

KEY WORDS

nursing process
assessment
nursing diagnosis
actual nursing diagnosis
risk nursing diagnosis
wellness nursing diagnosis
defining characteristics
medical diagnosis
collaborative problem
focused assessment
priority setting
measurable goal
   statements
nursing actions
nursing interventions
nursing orders
anticipated therapeutic
   outcomes

nursing interventions and
   implementation
nursing actions
dependent actions
interdependent actions
independent actions
drug history
primary sources
subjective data
secondary sources
tertiary sources
drug monographs
side effects
pathophysiology
therapeutic intent
side effects to report
side effects to expect

ASSIGNMENTS

Read textbook, pp. 23-41.
Study Review Sheets, Chapter 4.
Study Key Words associated with chapter content.
Complete Collaborative Activity.
Complete Practice Quiz.
Complete Chapter 4 Exam.

COLLABORATIVE ACTIVITY

Complete the following activity to prepare for in-class discussion and group work that may be assigned by the instructor.

After reading the section "Nursing Process for Nausea and Vomiting," Chapter 31, pp. 411 and 413, identify the specific questions that could be used to gather data to develop an individualized care plan for a patient who is experiencing nausea and vomiting during pregnancy. Add additional questions appropriate to the person and situation.

Copyright © 2001 by Mosby, Inc.   All rights reserved.

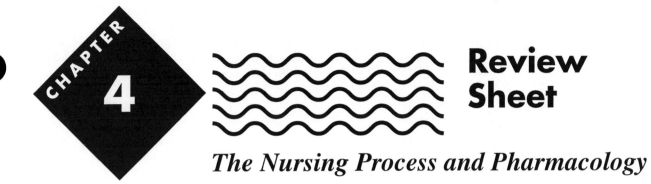

Review Sheet

The Nursing Process and Pharmacology

The QUESTION column and the ANSWER column have been offset so that you can cover the answer while reading the question, allowing you to assess your knowledge.

Question

1. Define *nursing diagnosis*.
2. State the five steps of the nursing process.

3. Explain the purpose of the assessment phase of the nursing process.

4. What are defining characteristics?

5. How does a medical diagnosis differ from a nursing diagnosis?

6. What is a collaborative problem?

7. Why is a focused assessment beneficial to the nurse?

8. Differentiate between an actual, risk, and possible nursing diagnosis.

9. What are the four phases of the planning process used to prepare to provide patient care?
10. Use Maslow's hierarchy of needs on p. 31 of the text to label the following individual needs and prioritize them according to importance: a) need for family visitors, b) need to avoid falls while ambulating, c) need for basic care to prevent skin breakdown, d) need for praise for learning about self-care.

Answer

1. A nursing diagnosis is a problem-solving method used in nursing.
2. The five steps of the nursing process are assessment, nursing diagnosis, planning, implementation, and evaluation.
3. Assessment is an ongoing data gathering process used to identify existing (actual) patient problems and/or to identify patient problems that may be evolving.
4. Defining characteristics are existing signs and symptoms that help define the presence of a patient problem. They provide clinical evidence of an existing or developing patient problem.
5. A medical diagnosis is a statement relating to a disease or disorder effect on the individual's physiological functioning. A nursing diagnosis defines a patient problem in which the nurse can intervene.
6. Collaborative problems require both medical or dental prescriptive orders and nursing interventions to monitor and evaluate the existing condition.
7. After establishing that a patient problem may or does exist, a focused assessment allows the nurse to concentrate the data collection process on a specific area that would help to define, validate, or negate the existence of a specific nursing diagnosis.
8. See definitions in textbook, pp. 27.

9. Planning encompasses: a) setting priorities, b) developing measurable goal statements, c) formulating nursing interventions, and d) developing anticipated therapeutic outcomes as a basis for evaluating the patient's status.

Copyright © 2001 by Mosby, Inc. All rights reserved.

11. Which of the following are nursing actions?
    a. giving a bed bath
    b. forcing fluids
    c. taking vital signs
    d. developing a medical diagnosis statement
12. Label the following nursing actions as "D" for dependent, "I" for interdependent, and "ID" for independent:
    a. administering a tube feeding
    b. administering prn medications
    c. positioning patient for comfort
    d. providing oral hygiene
    e. monitoring respiratory function between treatments by respiratory therapist
13. Develop a short-term goal for a patient receiving Maalox.

14. Explain why a drug history may be beneficial.

15. Label the following statements "S" for subjective data or "O" for objective data.
    a. "My medication makes me dizzy."
    b. "Yesterday the pain medication gave me good pain relief."
    c. One hour after administration of chemotherapy the nurse charts, "Patient vomited 4 ounces greenish-tinged, watery vomitus."
16. Turn to a drug classification section in the textbook. Find the area labeled Nursing Diagnosis. Explain the difference between indications and side effects when used to designate the nursing diagnoses associated with drug therapy.
17. Develop a statement for the therapeutic intent of a sedative for a patient having surgery tomorrow morning.

18. Differentiate between side effects to expect and side effects to report.

19. List common laboratory studies used to evaluate liver (hepatic) function and those used to evaluate kidney (renal) function.

20. When are culture and sensitivity (C&S) test taken?

10. During a period of ambulation, these needs would be in the following order: b, c, a, d. The priority could vary depending on variables present.

11. a, b, and c are nursing actions.

12. A and B are dependent, C and D are independent, and E is interdependent. Note: D could be dependent if the oral hygiene was specifically ordered by the physician.

13. Multiple possible answers. One example is: The patient will be able to state the correct schedule for self-administration of Maalox on Tuesday, (date).

14. A drug history can be used to identify current drugs, OTC and herbal products, being taken or problems relating to drug therapy, and to evaluate the need for medications.

15. A and B are subjective; C is objective.

16. Indications are nursing diagnosis statements that exist as a result of patient problems being experienced due to disruption of normal functioning by a disease process or disorder. Side effects are patient problems that have evolved as a result of drug therapy.

17. Therapeutic intent is to "provide rest and relaxation prior to surgery."

18. Side effects to expect are those that can generally be anticipated when the drug therapy is prescribed. It is important for the nurse to teach the patient steps he/she can take to minimize the side effects to make the drug therapy more tolerable. Side effects to report, also known as adverse drug effects, are those that require notification of the physician regarding the drug's action.

19. Hepatic function tests include AST, ALT, alkaline phosphatase, LDH, and GGT. Renal function tests include serum creatinine, creatinine clearance, blood urea nitrogen (BUN), and urinalysis.

 Copyright © 2001 by Mosby, Inc. All rights reserved.

21. What changes in the baseline CBC report should be reported to the physician?

22. Why are serum drug levels monitored?

23. What patient education should be done prior to discharge for all persons with medications prescribed?

24. List a minimum of five drugs that can be monitored by a blood draw.

20. C&S specimens (e.g., throat culture) are usually obtained prior to initiation of antibiotic therapy for an infection.

21. Elevated WBCs, bands, "segs," and/or lymphocytes should be reported.

22. Serum drug levels are monitored to establish whether the serum blood level of the specific drug is too low or in the nontherapeutic range, within the normal range and therapeutic, or too high and toxic to the patient.

23. Patient education before discharge should include drug name, dosage, route, and specific time(s) of administration; reason for taking the drug (therapeutic outcome or intent); side effects to expect and ways these can be minimized or eliminated; side effects to report; what to do if a dose is missed; and how to have the medication prescription filled.

24. Digoxin, theophylline, gentamicin, tobramycin, lithium, lidocaine, phenytoin, procainamide, quinidine, vancomycin, cyclosporine, and chloramphenicol can be monitored by a blood draw.

Copyright © 2001 by Mosby, Inc.   All rights reserved.

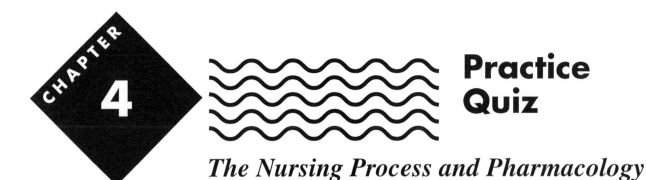

COMPLETION

Complete the following statements using key words from Chapter 4.

1. Mary tells you she developed nausea and vomiting four hours after taking the first dose of her newly prescribed antibiotic. This would be an example of (subjective, objective) data.

2. The nursing instructor tells the student nurse to collect further data relating to this case. The collection of patient data is known as the _____ phase of the nursing process.

3. Further inquiry reveals that Mary took the antibiotic on an empty stomach. In addition to gaining further information about the nausea and vomiting, the student nurse also asks Mary to tell her of all other medications being taken, both prescription and nonprescription. This is known as taking a(n) _____. Mary indicates that she does not regularly take any other medicine.

4. After collecting the data, the student reviews the drug monograph on the antibiotic. It states that nausea and vomiting are side effects to expect if taken on an empty stomach. The student nurse compares the signs and symptoms present with the _____ listed in a nursing diagnosis resource book to establish the _____.

5. Rescheduling of the time the medication is taken is an example of a nursing _____. The student nurse suggests that Mary take the next dose of the medication with food.

6. Based on the data assembled, the student nurse develops the following statement: Mary will self-administer the prescribed antibiotic with food at 6 A.M., 12 noon, 6 P.M., and midnight starting with the next dose. This is a _____ statement.

7. You notice on the physician's order sheet that a lab draw is ordered for gentamicin sulfate for a patient that was assigned to you. Important information for the laboratory to know is _____.

8. When a culture and sensitivity is ordered on a patient it is important to be sure the test is performed _____ the first dose of medication is administered.

9. Nursing diagnosis statements dealing with a patient with a family history of a disease who is likely to develop the disease would be called _____ nursing diagnosis statements.

Copyright © 2001 by Mosby, Inc.   All rights reserved.

Syllabus

Patient Education and Health Promotion

CHAPTER CONTENT

The Three Domains of Learning (p. 42)
Principles of Learning (p. 42)
Patient Education Associated with Medication Therapy
     (p. 46)

CHAPTER OBJECTIVES

The Three Domains of Learning

1. Differentiate the meanings of *cognitive, affective*, and *psychomotor learning*.
2. Identify the main principles of learning that must be applied during the teaching of a patient, family, or group.
3. Apply the principles of learning to the information learned in pharmacology.

Patient Education Associated with Medication Therapy

1. Describe essential elements of patient education in relation to the prescribed medications.
2. Describe the nurse's role in fostering patient responsibility for the maintenance of well-being and for compliance with the therapeutic regimen.
3. Identify the types of information that should be discussed with the patient or significant others in order to establish reasonable expectations for the prescribed therapy.
4. Discuss specific techniques used in the practice setting to document the patient education performed and degree of achievement attained.

KEY WORDS

cognitive domain
affective domain
psychomotor domain
objectives
ethnocentrism

scientific-biomedical
     paradigm
magicoreligious paradigm
holistic paradigm

ASSIGNMENTS

Read textbook pp. 41-48.
Study Key Words associated with the chapter content.
Complete Collaborative Activity as assigned.
Complete Chapter 5 Practice Quiz.
Complete Chapter 5 Exam.

COLLABORATIVE ACTIVITY

Complete the following activities to prepare for in-class discussion and group work that may be assigned by the instructor.

Preparing for interview:

1. Read Chapter 5.
2. Go to the library and find two articles on health teaching, preferably relating to pharmacology. Read and analyze the articles for additional ideas on health teaching that might benefit you.
3. Research recommended safe storage of medications in the home and available resources in the immediate area should an inadvertent poisoning occur.
4. Ask a friend, neighbor, or family member to participate in an interview regarding the medications currently being taken. Include both prescribed medications and over-the-counter (OTC) medicines. Stress that *NO* advice will be given regarding the medications, that this is strictly a data-gathering activity.
5. In accordance with school policy, have appropriate release forms signed prior to initiating the interview.

Purpose of interview:

The student will gain experience in data collection relating to medications. The data assembled will continue to be analyzed as the course progresses. For example, the administration techniques the individual describes for self-administration can be researched and analyzed during the study of medication administration.

Copyright © 2001 by Mosby, Inc.   All rights reserved.

Interview:

1. Explain the purpose of the interview and stress that no medical advice will be given regarding the medications discussed.
2. Take notes including the following information:
   a. In what type of environment was the interview conducted?
   b. List the medicines being taken by the interviewee, including those that have been prescribed by a physician as well as those purchased over-the-counter.
   c. For each drug discussed (a minimum of three) note the following:
      1) Name of drug
      2) Purpose for taking drug
      3) Length of time the drug(s) have been taken (e.g., one week, two years)
      4) Instructions given regarding how or when to discontinue the medicines (e.g., "take until the entire prescription is finished")
      5) Importance of taking these drugs as prescribed
      6) Any annoying symptoms experienced since starting on the medications and what has been done to relieve them
      7) Time schedule used when taking these medicines
      8) Self-administration techniques used when taking the medications
      9) Where the drugs are stored in the household
3. If the interviewee has questions regarding the medications, suggest discussing them with the physician or pharmacist.

Note to Student: It might be nice to send a "thank you" note to the participant following the interview.

Data analysis after the interview:

The data gathered during this interview will continue to be used as the course progresses and the student gains more knowledge of the study of pharmacology.

1. For each drug listed, state the generic and brand names.
2. Examine the drug monographs for the drugs listed. What are the anticipated therapeutic outcomes of these medicines? How does the information in the drug monograph correlate with the data provided by the interviewee?
3. Based on the length of time the drug has been taken, is it possible that drug tolerance may have occurred?
4. Read each drug monograph. Do any of the medicines being taken require gradual withdrawal upon discontinuation? What instructions should be given regarding the scheduling of the dosages? Was the time schedule the interviewee described appropriate for the medicine being taken?
5. What perception does the individual have of the importance of the medicines to the condition for which the medicines were prescribed? In the interviewee's opinion, are the medications important to the overall treatment of the condition?
6. What side effects to expect and side effects to report are listed for each drug in the monograph? Did the interviewee experience any of these? If so, were the actions used to minimize them appropriate?
7. Were the techniques of self-administration appropriate and accurate? If not, what changes should be suggested?
8. Based on the data collected, what nursing diagnosis statements are appropriate for the individual interviewed?
9. Establish goals and a health teaching plan for the person interviewed.
10. Was the person interviewed anxious to learn more about his/her medications? If so, how could you be of assistance?
11. Were drugs stored safely in the home setting? What suggestions could be made to improve the storage of or access to the medications?

Copyright © 2001 by Mosby, Inc.   All rights reserved.

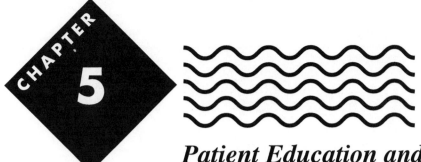

CHAPTER 5

Practice Quiz

Patient Education and Health Promotion

TRUE OR FALSE

Mark "T" for true or "F" for false for each statement.
<u>*Correct all false statements*</u>.

_____ 1. Explaining the various self-care needs to an individual and exploring his/her prior knowledge is an example of the affective domain learning.

_____ 2. Establishing an environment that is conducive to learning is essential to the overall learning process.

_____ 3. Deciding what to teach and how much to teach is essential to the learning process.

_____ 4. Utilizing an established teaching plan that all nurses can build on is important to the continuity of health teaching.

_____ 5. Health teaching is valued by all individuals equally.

_____ 6. Children may need adaptations in prepared learning materials based on their age, learning capabilities, and development.

_____ 7. It is best to explain all of the information needed for self-care so the teaching plan on the chart documents that all the health teaching was accomplished prior to discharge.

_____ 8. The magicoreligious belief system stresses that humans are under control of supernatural forces.

_____ 9. The scientific-biomedical belief system emphasizes health promotion and restoration.

_____ 10. Illness may not have the same meaning for all individuals.

Copyright © 2001 by Mosby, Inc.   All rights reserved.

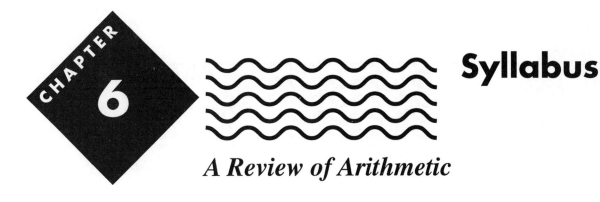

CHAPTER 6

A Review of Arithmetic

Syllabus

CHAPTER CONTENTS

Roman numerals (p. 49)
Fractions (p. 50)
Decimal fractions (p. 54)
Percents (p. 55)
Ratios (p. 56)
Systems of weights and measures (p. 57)
Calculation of intravenous fluid and medication rates (p. 63)
Fahrenheit and centigrade temperatures (p. 65)

CHAPTER OBJECTIVES

Roman Numerals

1. Read and write selected numerical values using Roman numerals.

Fractions

1. Demonstrate proficiency in calculating mathematical problems using addition, subtraction, multiplication, and/or division of fractions.

Decimal Fractions

1. Demonstrate proficiency in calculating mathematical problems using the addition, subtraction, multiplication, and/or division of decimals.
2. Convert decimals to fractions and fractions to decimals.

Percents

1. Demonstrate proficiency in calculating mathematical problems using percents.
2. Convert percents to fractions, percents to decimals, decimal fractions to percents, and common fractions to percents.

Ratios

1. Demonstrate proficiency in converting ratios to percents and percentages to ratios, in simplifying ratios, and in using the proportion method for solving problems.

Systems of Weights and Measures

1. Memorize the basic equivalents of the household, apothecary, and metric systems.
2. Demonstrate proficiency in performing conversion of medication problems utilizing the household, apothecary, and metric systems.

Calculation of Intravenous Fluid and Medication Rates

1. Use formulas to calculate intravenous fluid and medicine administration rates.

Fahrenheit and Centigrade (Celsius) Temperatures

1. Demonstrate proficiency in performing conversions between the centigrade and Fahrenheit systems of temperature measurement.

KEY WORDS

numerator	gram
denominator	administration sets
household measurements	drip chamber
apothecary measurements	macrodrip
grain	microdrip
minim	drop factor
milliliter	rounding
centimeter	centigrade
metric system	Fahrenheit
liter	Celsius

ASSIGNMENTS

Read textbook pages 49-66.
Complete Practice Quiz Parts 1 and 2, for Chapter 6.
Complete Chapter 6 Exam.

Copyright © 2001 by Mosby, Inc.   All rights reserved.

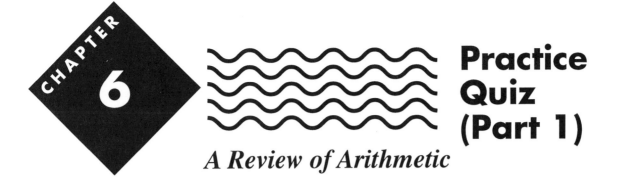

EQUIVALENTS AND CONVERSION

Memorize the equivalents listed in Chapter 6 then do the following self-test. Write the answer in the blank provided.

Household Equivalents

1. 4 cups = _____ quarts
2. 1 tablespoon = _____ teaspoons
3. 8 ounces = _____ cup(s)
4. 1 pint = _____ cup(s)

Apothecary Equivalents

5. 1 fluid dram = _____ ml
6. 8 fluid drams = _____ fluid ounces
7. 8 drams = _____ grains
8. 1 dram = _____ grains

Metric Equivalents

9. 1 ml = _____ cc
10. 1 liter = _____ ml
11. 1 milligram (mg) = _____ micrograms (μg)
12. 1 gram (g) = _____ milligrams (mg)
13. 1 gram (g) = _____ grains (gr)

Conversion Rules

14. To convert grams to grains: _____.
15. To convert grains to grams: _____.
16. To convert milligrams to grams: _____.
17. To convert grains to milligrams:_____.

STOP! IF YOU HAVE NOT MEMORIZED THE EQUIVALENTS AND THE CONVERSION RULES YOU SHOULD NOT PROCEED UNTIL YOU HAVE DONE SO.

Copyright © 2001 by Mosby, Inc.   All rights reserved.

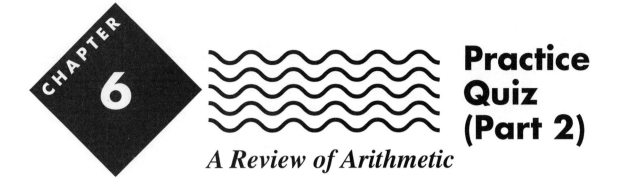

Practice Quiz (Part 2)

A Review of Arithmetic

ROMAN NUMERALS

Convert the following Arabic numerals to Roman numerals.

1. 5   = _____
2. 7 1/2 = _____
3. 4   = _____
4. 15   = _____
5. 20   = _____
6. 24   = _____

FRACTIONS

Identify the numerator or denominator for each of the following fractions as indicated.

7. 1/5   numerator is _____
8. 2/3   numerator is _____
9. 3/8   numerator is _____
10. 1 1/2   denominator is _____
11. 9/10   denominator is _____
12. 2 2/5   numerator is _____
13. 6/10   denominator is _____
14. 1 1/3   denominator is _____

Which of the following fractions is the largest? Circle your answer.

15. 1/8 or 1/16
16. 2/3 or 3/4
17. 1/100 or 1/200
18. 1/4 or 1/3
19. 3/8 or 7/8
20. 1/150 or 1/90

Reduce the following fractions.

21. 4/16   = _____
22. 12/24   = _____
23. 4/8   = _____
24. 36/48   = _____
25. 1 12/18   = _____
26. 3 34/85   = _____
27. 1 6/8   = _____
28. 12 6/8   = _____
29. 2 30/60   = _____
30. 3/9   = _____

Write the following fractions as decimals. When applicable, carry decimal to thousandths and round to <u>hundredths</u>.

31. 7/8   = _____
32. 5/6   = _____
33. 1 3/4 = _____
34. 2/3   = _____
35. 15/16 = _____
36. 1/3   = _____
37. 5/8   = _____
38. 7/9   = _____
39. 1/16   = _____
40. 1/2   = _____

Multiply the following fractions. Reduce answers to lowest terms.

41. 1/3 x 1/4=
42. 2/3 x 3/8=
43. 7/8 x 1/2=
44. 3/4 x 7/8=
45. 1/2 x 4/7=
46. 7/8 x 2/3=
47. 1 1/2 x 3/4=
48. 2 2/3 x 4/5=

Divide the following. As appropriate, carry to hundredths and round to <u>tenths</u>.

49. 2/3 ÷ 7/8=
50. 1/3 ÷ 1/2=
51. 5/9 ÷ 1/4=
52. 21.78 ÷ 1.23=
53. 756 ÷ 12.3=
54. 32 ÷ 1.78=
55. 112 ÷ .06=
56. 1.22 ÷ .32=
57. 3.789 ÷ .112=

Change the following percents to decimals and the fractions to percents.

58. 56%   = _____
59. 1/150 = _____%
60. 2/3   = _____%
61. 75%   = _____
62. 1/2% = _____

Copyright © 2001 by Mosby, Inc.   All rights reserved.

63. 3/4   = _____%
64. 7/8   = _____%
65. 123% = _____

Change the following decimals to fractions and the fractions to decimals.

66. 0.3   = _____
67. .003   = _____
68. .03   = _____
69. 4/10   = _____
70. 4/100 = _____
71. 4/1000 = _____

DIRECTIONS: Change the following percents to ratios.

72. 75%   = _____
73. 60%   = _____
74. 1/2% = _____

Convert the following using equivalency tables.

75. 1 quart = _____ cup(s)
76. _____ ounces = 1 pint
77. 3 teaspoon = _____ tablespoon(s)
78. 2 g = _____ gr
79. .125 g = _____ mg
80. 6 gr = _____ mg
81. 250 mg = _____ g
82. 1 fl dram = _____ ml
83. 1 teaspoon = _____ ml
84. 6 lbs = _____ Kg (round to hundredths)
85. 165 lbs = _____ Kg

Copyright © 2001 by Mosby, Inc.   All rights reserved.

CHAPTER CONTENTS

CHAPTER OBJECTIVES

Legal and Ethical Considerations

1. Research the Nurse Practice Act in the state where you are practicing. Identify the limitations relating to medication administration placed on licensed practical/vocational nurses, registered nurses, and nurse clinicians.
2. Study the policies and procedures of the practice setting to identify specific regulations concerning medication administration by licensed practical/vocational nurses, registered nurses, and nurse clinicians.

Patient Charts

1. Identify the basic categories of information available in a patient's chart.
2. Study the patient charts at different practice settings to identify the various formats used to chart patient data.
3. Cite the information contained in a Kardex and describe the purpose of this file.

Drug Distribution Systems

1. Cite the advantages and disadvantages of the ward stock system, the computer-controlled dispensing system, the individual prescription order system, and the unit dose system of drug distribution.
2. Study the narcotic control system used at your assigned clinical practice setting and compare it to the requirements of the Controlled Substance Act of 1970.

The Drug Order

1. Define the four categories of medication orders used.

2. Describe the procedure used in your assigned clinical setting for taking, recording, transcribing, and verifying verbal medication orders.

The Six Rights of Drug Administration

1. Identify specific precautions needed to ensure that the right drug is prepared for the patient.
2. Memorize and recite standard abbreviations associated with the scheduling of medications.
3. Identify data found in the patient's chart that must be analyzed to determine if the patient has abnormal renal or hepatic function.
4. Describe specific safety precautions the nurse should follow to ensure that correct medication calculations are performed.
5. Review the policies and procedures of your practice setting to identify drugs the dosages of which must be checked by two qualified persons.
6. Describe the methods that should be used to ensure that the correct patient receives the correct medication, by the correct route, in the correct amount, at the correct time.
7. Compare each safety measure for preparation and administration of medications described in the text with those procedures used at your clinical practice setting.
8. Identify appropriate nursing actions for documenting the administration and therapeutic effectiveness of each medication administered.

KEY WORDS

Nurse Practice Act
summary sheet
physician's order form
flow sheet
consent form
graphic record
history and physical
   examination form
progress notes
nurse's notes

prn medication record
nursing admission
   assessment
critical pathways or case
   management plan
nursing care plan
laboratory tests record
other diagnostic tests
consultation reports

Copyright © 2001 by Mosby, Inc.   All rights reserved.

medication administration
   record (MAR)
Kardex records
patient education record
ward stock system
computer-controlled
   dispensing system
individual prescription
   system

unit dose system
long-term care unit dose
   system
stat orders
standing orders
renewal orders
prn order
verification
transcription

ASSIGNMENTS

Read textbook pages 67-84.
Study Key Words associated with chapter content.
Complete Practice Quiz Chapter 7.
Complete Collaborative Activities for Chapter 7.
Complete Chapter 7 Exam.

COLLABORATIVE ACTIVITY

Complete the following activities to prepare for in-class discussion and group work that may be assigned by the instructor.

1. Research how drug orders are taken and transcribed in the clinical sites where you are assigned. Include rules for orders that are received by fax.
2. Charting Exercise
   a. What time frames are used in the clinical site where assigned when drugs are ordered?

Abbreviation	*Timeframe*
bid	
tid	
ac	
pc	
qid	
q 4 h	
q 6 h	
hs	

b. Use the MAR record on the next page and other forms as appropriate from a clinical site where assigned to transcribe the following orders. Use military time and the customary time frames for medication scheduling.

Chart for: Martha Washburn
                 1616 Tangerine Blvd.
                 Hometown, Pa.
                 Rm.454—Bed 2
                 Patient No. 123456
                 Dr. Ballantyne

Physician's Order Form

Date:	*Time:*	*Physician's Order:*	*Doctor:*
Today	0700	acebutolol 400 mg po, bid	
		acetaminophen 600 mg po,	
		q3h, prn temperature	
		> 101.6 °F	
		cefadroxil 1000 mg po, bid	
		MOM 30 ml daily	
		prn constipation	
		Signed by Dr. Ballantyne	

Copyright © 2001 by Mosby, Inc.   All rights reserved.

MARTINDALE HOMETOWN HOSPITAL

MEDICATION ADMINISTRATION RECORD

NAME:	RM-BD:	Init Signature Title
ID NO.:	AGE:	
DIAGNOSIS:	SEX:	

PHYSICIAN:	Ht:	Wt:

SCHEDULED MEDICATIONS

DATE	MEDICATION-STRENGTH-FORM-ROUTE	0030-0729	0730-1529	1530-0029

** PRN MEDICATIONS**

Copyright © 2001 by Mosby, Inc.   All rights reserved.

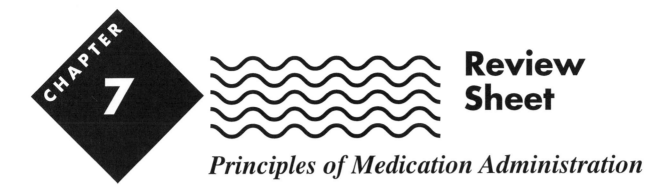

Review Sheet

Principles of Medication Administration

The QUESTION column and the ANSWER column have been offset so that you can cover the answer while reading the question, allowing you to assess your knowledge.

Questions	Answers
1. Can an employing agency write policies that require the nurse to exceed the standards established by the state board of nursing/nursing licensing agency?	
2. What types of medications may have restrictions regarding the qualifications of an individual to administer the medicine?	1. No. Policies of the employing agency can authorize less than, but not more than, the established maximum standards.
3. What information is the nurse expected to know about a specific drug before administering it?	2. Antineoplastic medicines, Imferon, RhoGAM, allergy extracts, and heparin are administered in accordance with specific limitations of the employing agency. Most policies require doses of heparin and insulin to be checked by two qualified individuals.
4. What information should be recorded whenever a "prn" medicine is to be administered?	3. See textbook, p. 67.
5. Examine the sections on a medication administration record (MAR) to identify the categories used.	4. Date, time, drug name, dose, route of administration, reason for administration and the patient's response to the medication.
6. Where would information regarding a patient's possible allergies be found?	5. Medication administration records are usually divided into four sections: scheduled section, parenteral section, stat section, and prn medication section.
7. Explain the differences between the ward stock, computer-controlled, individual prescription order, and unit dose drug distribution (acute and long-term care) systems.	6. Information about a patient's allergies is recorded in the history and physical section of the chart, the Kardex, the MAR, the patient's chart holder, and on the patient's allergy bracelet.
8. Referring to the narcotic substance inventory form, Figure 7-12, list narcotic drugs routinely used in the acute care setting.	7. See textbook, pp. 77-79.
9. What information is recorded on the controlled substance inventory form when a controlled substance is administered?	8. See Figure 7-12, p. 79.

Copyright © 2001 by Mosby, Inc.   All rights reserved.

10. Explain the differences between a stat order, standing order, prn order, verbal order, and fax order.

11. How is a drug order verified and transcribed?
12. What are the six RIGHTS of drug administration?
13. What tests are used to identify hepatic and renal function?

14. What methods are used to ensure correct identification of a patient prior to drug administration? (Discuss adults, children, and inpatient and outpatient settings.)

15. Review commonly used abbreviations for the scheduling of medication administration.

9. The date, time, name of medicine administered, patient's name, amount wasted (if any), and the number of dosage containers (such as unit dose tablets or ampoules) remaining after the drug is removed. The nurse administering the medicine signs the record as well as the qualified witness if any medicine is wasted.

10. See textbook, pp. 80-81.
11. See textbook, p. 81.
12. The six rights of drug administration are: Right Drug, Right Time, Right Dose, Right Patient, Right Route, and Right Documentation.
13. Liver function tests include aspartate aminotransferase (AST), alanine aminotransferase (ALT), alkaline phosphatase, lactic dehydrogenase (LDH), and gamma glutamyl transferase (GGT). Renal function tests include serum creatinine, creatinine clearance, blood urea nitrogen, and urinalysis.
14. See textbook, p. 83.

15. See textbook Appendix A, Prescription Abgreviations.

Copyright © 2001 by Mosby, Inc.   All rights reserved.

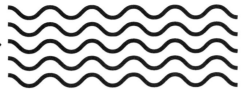

Practice Quiz

Principles of Medication Administration

MATCHING

Match the definition with the corresponding term.

_____ 1. prn medications
_____ 2. physician's order form
_____ 3. MAR
_____ 4. "stat"
_____ 5. Kardex

a. Check this section of the patient chart when questioning details of a drug order on the MAR.
b. Give around the clock.
c. Give immediately.
d. Administer as required or necessary within defined limits of drug order.
e. Record scheduled drugs administered here.
ab. Section of the patient record containing the care plan.
ac. Controlled substances are recorded here when administered.

MULTIPLE CHOICE

Select the BEST answer and write the letter selected in the space provided.

_____ 6. 6 A.M. in military time is
    a. 0600.
    b. 1200.
    c. 1800.
    d. 2200.

_____ 7. 2 P.M. in military time is
    a. 0200.
    b. 0600.
    c. 1200.
    d. 1400.

_____ 8. The inventory control record is completed when the
    a. patient asks for a controlled substance.
    b. controlled substance is removed.
    c. medication is administered.
    d. degree of pain relief is assessed.

_____ 9. The prn medication record is completed
    a. when the patient asks for a controlled substance.
    b. when the controlled substance is removed.
    c. immediately after administering the drug.
    d. when the degree of pain relief is assessed.

_____ 10. The narcotic control count is performed by
    a. the charge nurse.
    b. a nurse going off duty.
    c. a nurse coming on duty.
    d. two nurses; one from shift going off duty and one from shift coming on duty.

_____ 11. A drug on a scheduled order is given
    a. as many times as needed.
    b. at prescribed/designated intervals.
    c. one time only.
    d. immediately.

_____ 12. A student nurse may accept a verbal drug order.
    a. true
    b. false

_____ 13. When a verbal order is taken it must be co-signed and dated by the physician within
    a. 3 days.
    b. 2 days.
    c. 24 hours.
    d. 12 hours.

_____ 14. The person responsible for the transcription of the drug order is the
    a. nurse's aide.
    b. unit secretary/ward clerk.
    c. physician.
    d. nurse.

 Copyright © 2001 by Mosby, Inc. All rights reserved.

_____ 15. When "wasting" a portion of a dose of narcotic, the nurse must have this witnessed by
   a. the prescribing physician.
   b. the charge nurse.
   c. a second qualified nurse.
   d. the medication aide.

_____ 16. When measuring a fractional dose of a medication with a volume of less than 1 ml, the most accurate method would be to use a
   a. medicine cup.
   b. tuberculin syringe.
   c. teaspoon.
   d. medicine dropper.

_____ 17. The most reliable method of calculating pediatric drug doses is using _____.
   a. body surface area (BSA)
   b. Clark's rule
   c. a fraction of the adult dose
   d. Pyxis system of measurement

_____ 18. A client has a new drug ordered bid. This means the drug will be administered
   a. once daily.
   b. two times per day.
   c. three times per day.
   d. four times per day.

_____ 19. The Pyxis system refers to a(n)
   a. narcotic inventory system.
   b. individual prescription order system.
   c. unit dose system used primarily in long-term care.
   d. electronic medication dispensing system.

_____ 20. The medication administration record (MAR) in a long-term care setting is designed to be used for
   a. 8 hours.
   b. 24 hours.
   c. 1 week.
   d. 1 month.

ESSAY

21. What information is included on a written prescription?

22. Explain the procedure used to check the drug name against the drug order during the preparation of medications.

Copyright © 2001 by Mosby, Inc.   All rights reserved.

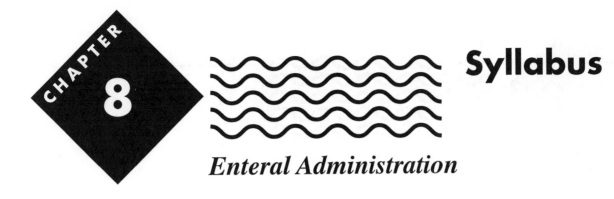

CHAPTER 8

Syllabus

Enteral Administration

CHAPTER CONTENTS

Administration of Oral Medications (p. 85)
Administration of Solid-Form Oral Medications (p. 88)
Administration of Liquid-Form Oral Medications (p. 90)
Administration of Medications by Nasogastric Tube
    (p. 92)
Administration of Enteral Feedings (p. 94)
Administration of Rectal Suppositories (p. 96)
Administration of a Disposable Enema (p. 97)

CHAPTER OBJECTIVES

Administration of Oral Medications

1. Correctly define and identify oral dosage forms of medications.
2. Identify common receptacles used to administer oral medications.

Administration of Solid-Form Oral Medications

1. Describe general principles of administering solid forms of medications and the different techniques utilized with a medication card, computer-controlled, and unit dose distribution systems.

Administration of Liquid-Form Oral Medications

1. Compare techniques used to administer liquid forms of oral medications utilizing medication card and unit dose systems of distribution.

Administration of Medications by Nasogastric Tube

1. Cite the equipment needed, techniques used, and precautions necessary when administering medications via a nasogastric tube.

Administration of Enteral Feedings

1. Discuss ways to meet a person's basic metabolic requirements and provide adequate nutritional intake through the use of enteral nutrition support.

Administration of Rectal Suppositories

1. Cite the equipment needed and techniques used to administer rectal suppositories.

Administration of a Disposable Enema

1. Cite the equipment needed and techniques used to administer a disposable enema.

KEY WORDS

capsules
lozenges
tablets
elixirs
emulsions
suspensions
syrups

unit dose package
souffle cup
medicine cup
medicine dropper
oral syringe
nasogastric tube

ASSIGNMENTS

Read textbook pages 85-98.
Study Key Words associated with the chapter content.
Complete Practice Quiz for Chapter 8.
Complete Practical Exam for Chapter 8.
Complete Written Exam for Chapter 8.

Copyright © 2001 by Mosby, Inc.   All rights reserved.

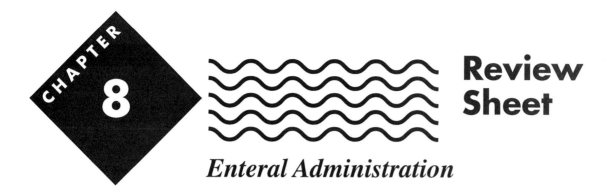

Enteral Administration

The Question column and the Answer column have been offset so that you can cover the answer while reading the question, allowing you to assess your knowledge.

Question	**Answer**
1. When an individual is unable to swallow or has had oral surgery, an alternative route of administration is the _____ route.	
2. A major advantage of using the rectal route for drug administration is _____.	1. nasogastric
3. List the composition and advantages of the following dosage forms: capsules, time-released capsules, lozenges, tablets, elixirs, emulsions, suspensions, and syrups.	2. bypass the digestive enzymes and avoid irritation to the stomach, esophagus, and stomach.
4. Why is it important to use the medicine dropper that accompanies a medication?	3. See textbook, pp. 85-86.
5. Why is an oral syringe preferred over a household teaspoon for administering a medication?	4. The dropper has been specifically made to correspond with the viscosity of the drug to deliver the correct volume of medication.
6. List the 5 RIGHTS of medication administration.	5. An oral syringe is more accurate.
7. What is the 6th RIGHT of medication administration and why is it important?	6. The five rights of drug administration are: RIGHT Patient, RIGHT Drug, RIGHT dosage, RIGHT time of administration, and RIGHT route of administration.
8. What are the primary principles of giving a solid form and liquid form of a medication?	7. RIGHT documentation explains not only what was administered but also the patient's response.
9. Discuss the proper method(s) of checking NG tube placement prior to the administration of a drug or an enteral formula.	8. See textbook, pp. 88-92.
10. Identify the color and pH values of gastric, intestinal, and pleural secretions both with and without the administration of H_2 blockers (antagonists).	9. Verify NG location after initial placement using x-ray verification BEFORE administering any drug or enteral formula for the first time. (See textbook, p. 93.)
11. Name four general categories of enteral formulas.	10. See textbook, Method 1: pH testing of gastric contents, p. 93.
12. How long can an enteral formula be left standing open with refrigeration?	11. Four general types of enteral formulas are intact (polymeric) nutrient, elemental, disease- or condition-specific, and modular nutrients.
13. Review the procedure for NG administration of enteral formulas using bolus and continuous infusion techniques.	12. An open enteral formula can be kept refrigerated up to 24 hours. The tubing and formula receptacle used for a continuous method of delivery such as the Kangaroo also should be changed every 24 hours.

Copyright © 2001 by Mosby, Inc.   All rights reserved.

14. State the positioning used for a patient when he/she is receiving an NG feeding using the bolus and using a continuous delivery method.

15. How are rectal suppositories inserted?

16. What position is the patient placed in to administer a disposable enema?

13. See textbook, pp. 92-96.

14. Place patient in semi-Fowler's position with head of bed (HOB) elevated 30 degrees for 30 minutes before and at least one hour after a bolus feeding. Most patients with a continuous feeding are maintained at a 30 to 45 degree elevation of the HOB.

15. Apply a glove or finger cot, have suppository in a solid form, use water-soluble lubricant or plain water to moisten, then insert suppository about one inch past the internal sphincter in the rectum.

16. To administer a disposable enema, place the patient on the left side.

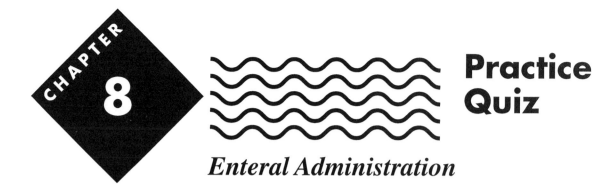

Practice Quiz

Enteral Administration

COMPLETION

Complete the following statements.

1. Capsules are _____.
2. Timed-release tablets differ from capsules by
   _____.
3. Lozenges or troches are administered by _____ route and patient should be instructed to
   _____.
4. Elixirs are drugs dissolved in _____.
5. Syrups are drugs dissolved in _____.
6. Emulsions and suspensions are similar in that
   _____ .
7. 1 oz (fl oz) on the medicine cup equals _____ Tbsp.
8. 1 tsp on the medicine cup equals _____ ml.

TRUE OR FALSE

Mark "T" for true or "F" for false for each question.
Correct all false statements.

_____ 9. The oral dropper that accompanied a specific drug is lost. The nurse should substitute a dropper from another medication for the lost one.

_____ 10. To validate the correct placement of a nasogastric (NG) tube prior to administering a medication or enteral feeding it is acceptable to aspirate gastric contents and check the pH and color.

_____ 11. When flushing an NG tube, do not clamp the tube until all the solution has time to reach the stomach.

_____ 12. When documenting an enteral feeding, the amount administered is charted on the intake and output sheet and then is included in the intake total for each shift.

_____ 13. Intermittent tube feedings require that the unused formula mixed and dispensed by the pharmacy be discarded every 48 hours.

_____ 14. The head of the bed (HOB) is elevated 30 minutes before and 30 minutes to 1 hour after administering an intermittent tube feeding.

_____ 15. Rectal suppositories are generally inserted with the patient positioned in the Sims' position.

_____ 16. A disposable enema is administered with the patient positioned on the right side.

_____ 17. When testing gastric pH for a person NOT taking an H_2 blocker, such as ranitidine, the gastric contents would have a pH of 1.0 to 4.0.

_____ 18. When testing gastric pH for a person who IS taking an H_2 blocker, such as ranitidine, the gastric contents would have a pH > 4.0.

_____ 19. Aspirated intestinal fluid should be a clear-to-straw colored secretion.

_____ 20. Auscultation is an accurate method of checking nasogastric tube placement.

Copyright © 2001 by Mosby, Inc.   All rights reserved.

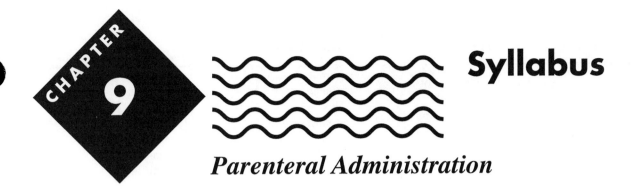

Syllabus

Parenteral Administration

CHAPTER CONTENTS

CHAPTER OBJECTIVES

Equipment Used in Parenteral Administration

1. Name the three parts of a syringe.
2. Read the calibrations of the cubic centimeter or milliliter scale on different types of syringes.
3. Read the volume of medication on a glass syringe and a plastic syringe.
4. Give examples of volumes of medications that can be measured in a tuberculin syringe, rather than a larger-volume syringe.
5. State the advantages and disadvantages of using prefilled syringes.
6. Explain the system of measurement utilized to define the inside diameter of a syringe.
7. Identify the parts of a needle.
8. Explain how the gauge of a needle is determined.
9. Compare the usual volume of medication that can be administered at one site by intradermal, subcutaneous, or intramuscular routes.
10. State the criteria used for the selection of the correct needle gauge and length.
11. Identify the parts of an intravenous administration set.
12. State where to find the number of drops per milliliter delivered by the drip chambers on intravenous administration sets purchased from different manufacturers.
13. Identify the meaning of needle protector systems.

Parenteral Dosage Forms

1. Differentiate among ampules, vials, and Mix-O-Vials.
2. Describe the different types of large-volume solution containers available.

Preparation of Parenteral Medication

1. List the equipment needed for the preparation of parenteral medications.
2. Describe, practice, and perfect the preparation of medications using the various dosage forms for parenteral administration.
3. Describe, practice, and perfect the technique of preparing two different drugs in one syringe, such as insulin or a preoperative medication.

Administration of Medication by the Intradermal Route

1. Identify the equipment needed and describe the technique used to administer a medication via the intradermal route.

Administration of Medication by the Subcutaneous Route

1. Identify the equipment needed and describe the technique used to administer a medication via the subcutaneous route.

Administration of Medication by the Intramuscular Route

1. Identify the equipment needed and describe the technique used to administer medications in the vastus lateralis muscle, rectus femoris muscle, ventrogluteal area, dorsogluteal area, or the deltoid muscle.
2. For each anatomical site studied, describe the landmarks used to identify the site before administration of the medication.
3. Identify good sites for intramuscular administration of medication in an infant, a child, an adult, and an elderly person.

Copyright © 2001 by Mosby, Inc. All rights reserved.

43

Administration of Medication by the Intravenous Route

1. Identify the dosage forms available, sites of administration, and general principles of administering medications via the intravenous route.
2. Describe the precautions needed to prevent the transmission of HIV that should be implemented for all patients requiring venipuncture.
3. Describe the correct techniques for administering medications via an established peripheral or central intravenous line, a vascular access device, a heparin lock, an intravenous bag, a bottle or volume-control device, or through a secondary piggyback set.
4. Describe the recommended guidelines and procedures for intravenous catheter care (including proper maintenance of patency of IV lines and implanted access device), IV line dressing changes, and for peripheral and central venous IV needle or catheter changes.
5. Discuss the proper baseline patient assessments needed to evaluate the intravenous therapy (e.g., phlebitis, extravasation, air in the tubing).
6. Review the policies and procedures used at the practice setting that ensure that persons performing venipunctures and intravenous therapy have the required proficiency.

KEY WORDS

barrel	anergic
plunger	erythema
tip	papules
minim scale	vesicles
milliliter scale	subcutaneous
insulin syringe	intramuscular
tuberculin syringe	vastus lateralis
prefilled syringe	rectus femoris
needle gauge	ventrogluteal
butterfly/winged needles	dorsogluteal area
ampule	deltoid muscle
vials	Z-track method
Mix-O-Vials	intravenous
tandem setup	venipuncture
piggyback	phlebitis
IV rider	infiltration
intradermal	pulmonary edema
wheal	pulmonary embolism

ASSIGNMENTS

Read textbook, pages 99-138.
Study Key Words associated with the chapter content.
Complete Practice Quiz, Chapter 9.
Complete the Practical Test, Chapter 9.
Complete Chapter 9 Exam.

Copyright © 2001 by Mosby, Inc.   All rights reserved.

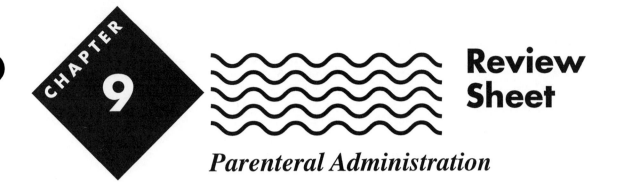

CHAPTER 9

Review Sheet

Parenteral Administration

The Question column and the Answer column have been offset so that you can cover the answer while reading the question, allowing you to assess your knowledge.

Question	Answer
1. Define *parenteral*.	1. Parenteral medication administration routes are intradermal, intramuscular (IM), and intravenous (IV) injections.
2. What are the major advantages of parenteral medication administration?	2. See textbook, p. 99.
3. List the parts of a syringe and the method of reading the measuring scale on the tuberculin, 3 ml, and insulin syringes.	3. Figures 9-4, 9-2, 9-3.
4. What volume can safely be injected at one site for intradermal, SC, IM, and IV medications?	4. See Table 9-1, p. 104.
5. The inner diameter of a needle is known as _____.	5. Gauge: the larger the number, the smaller the diameter.
6. Name the parts of an IV administration set.	6. See Figure 9-14, p. 106.
7. List the parts of an IV and the setup of a piggy-back.	7. See Figure 9-18, p. 108.
8. Discuss how needle sizes are selected for correct delivery of SC, IM, or IV medications.	8. Examine Figure 9-13, p. 105.
9. Differentiate between an ampule, a vial, and a Mix-O-Vial. Read section on removal of medications from these containers.	9. See textbook, pp. 106, 111, 113.
10. Describe the correct method of preparing two types of insulin in the same syringe.	10. See textbook Figure 9-23, p. 114.
11. List the terms associated with intradermal administration and reading of the reactions.	11. See textbook, pp. 115. 117.
12. Describe patient education that should be done in advance and at the time of performing intradermal testing.	12. See textbook, p. 116.
13. What types of subcutaneous injections do NOT require aspiration prior to injection of the medication?	13. Heparin and insulin do not require aspiration prior to injection.
14. List the injection sites used for IM injections.	14. See textbook, pp. 120-121.
15. Why is the gluteal area NOT used for IM injections in children under three years of age?	15. The gluteal muscle is not adequately developed.
16. When is the Z-track method of IM injection used?	

Copyright © 2001 by Mosby, Inc.   All rights reserved.

17. Identify common sites for starting an IV in an adult.

18. Identify common sites for starting an IV in a child.
19. What are vascular access devices?
20. Explain the SASH technique used during intravenous administration of medications.
21. What is a commonly accepted rate for a TKO (to keep open) IV order?

22. What is the purpose of performing a premedication assessment?
23. What is the formula used to calibrate the rate of an IV drip rate?

24. Discuss the correct setup for the administration of an IV piggyback medication.
25. Describe the correct method of monitoring a running IV.
26. Describe how to assess infiltration at an IV site.
27. If you see air in the tubing of a running IV, what should you do?

28. What are the signs and symptoms of circulatory overload and pulmonary edema?

16. The Z-track method is used with medications that are particularly irritating, or that will stain the skin (e.g. injectable iron)
17. See Figures 9-39 and 9-40, p. 127.
18. See Figure 9-41, p. 128.
19. These are implantable infusion ports that are used for long-term intravenous therapy. (See Figure 9-43.)
20. **S=** Saline
    A= Administer drug
    S= Saline
    H= Heparin (Not all types of vascular access devices require the use of heparin; check hospital policy.)
21. A commonly accepted rate for TKO IV is 10 ml/hr.

22. Premedication assessment is performed to prevent the administration of a medication to a patient whose diagnosis, symptoms, or other data indicate the medication should not be administered.
23. See textbook, p. 132.

24. See textbook, pp. 108, Figure 9-18.

25. See textbook, pp. 136-138.
26. Apply a tourniquet proximal to the infusion site to constrict flow. Continued flow with the tourniquet in place confirms infiltration.
27. Clamp the tubing; use a syringe to withdraw the air pocket.
28. Symptoms of circulatory overload include engorged neck veins, dyspnea, reduced urine output, edema, bounding pulse, shallow, and rapid respirations. Symptoms of pulmonary edema include dyspnea, cough, anxiety, rales, rhonchi, and frothy sputum.

Copyright © 2001 by Mosby, Inc.   All rights reserved.

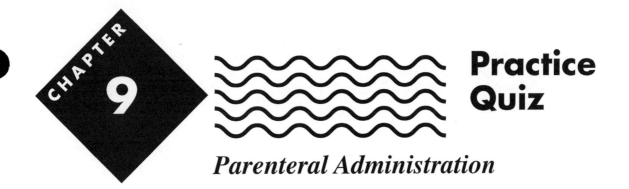

Study the chapter content then take the practice quiz to test your knowledge.

LABEL THE SYRINGE BELOW

1.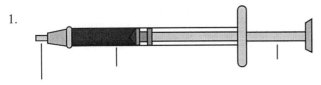

READ THE FOLLOWING SYRINGES

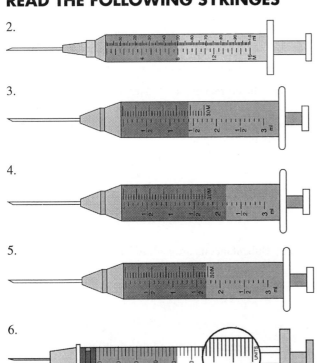

2.

3.

4.

5.

6.

7.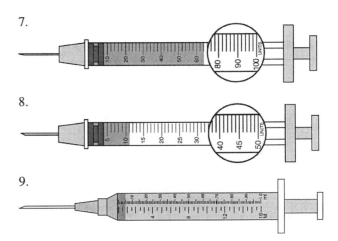

8.

9.

10.

11.

12.

LABEL THE PARTS OF A NEEDLE

13.

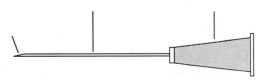

Copyright © 2001 by Mosby, Inc.   All rights reserved.

COMPLETION

In the blanks provided, write the volume of a drug that can be injected at one site by the following methods.

14. Intradermal: _____ ml
15. Subcutaneous: _____ ml
16. Intramuscular: _____ ml
    Divided dose is: _____
17. Intravenous fluid: _____ ml

PRACTICE INTRAVENOUS CALCULATIONS

18. Give 100 ml/hr 5% D/W using a 20 gtts/ml administration set. Run at _____ gtts/min.
19. Give 125 ml/hr lactated Ringer's using a 15 gtts/ml administration set. Run at _____ gtts/min.
20. Give 1000 ml 5% D/W over 10 hrs using a 10 gtts/ml administration set. Run at _____ gtts/min.
21. Give 250 ml 0.9% sodium chloride over 2 hours using a 15 gtts/ml administration set. Run at _____ gtts/min.

LABEL THE FOLLOWING

22. This is known as a(n) _____.

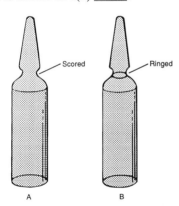

Explain how to withdraw fluid from this receptacle.

23. This is known as a(n) _____.

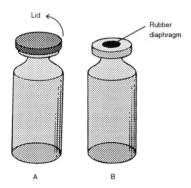

Explain how to withdraw fluid from this receptacle.

24. This is known as a(n) _____.

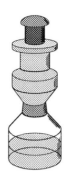

Explain how to withdraw fluid from this receptacle.

DRAW A DIAGRAM OF THE FOLLOWING

25. There are two bags of intravenous solution to be hung for the patient. One is a 1000 ml D5/W; the second is 100 ml 0.9% sodium chloride containing a medication. Draw how these would be arranged on the IV pole.

26. Draw the correct angle of insertion of a needle for each of the following types of injections. Include the dermis, epidermis, muscle, and subcutaneous tissue layers in the diagram.
    a. Intradermal drug administration:

    b. Subcutaneous drug administration:

    c. Intramuscular drug administration:

  Copyright © 2001 by Mosby, Inc.   All rights reserved.

27. Label the figure below with the injection sites used for subcutaneous drug administration.

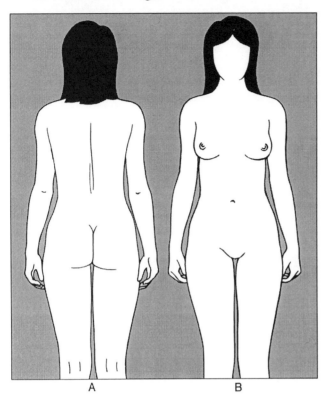

A   B

28. Draw a diagram to illustrate where an intramuscular injection is given to an adult in the vastus lateralis muscle. Include the following structures in the drawing: greater trochanter, femoral artery and vein, sciatic nerve, patella, and vastus lateralis muscle.

29. Draw a diagram to illustrate where an intramuscular injection is given to a child in the ventrogluteal site. Include the following structures in the drawing: iliac crest, anterior superior iliac spine, gluteus medius, and greater trochanter.

30. Label the pictures below with the sites for intramuscular injection in a child and an adult.

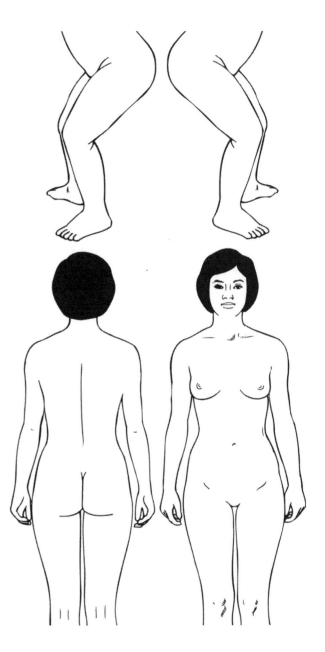

31. Draw positioning of a patient for an intramuscular injection into the dorsal gluteal site.

Copyright © 2001 by Mosby, Inc.   All rights reserved.

ESSAY

32. Explain how to prepare 22 U Regular and 15 U NPH insulin in a syringe.
    Note: Review: How many units of insulin = 1 cc?
33. What intravenous sites are commonly used in small children?
34. Explain the SASH routine for flushing IVs. Compare this with the procedure used at the clinical site where you are assigned.

 Copyright © 2001 by Mosby, Inc.   All rights reserved.

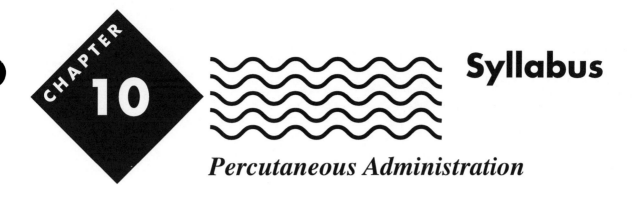

CHAPTER 10

Syllabus

Percutaneous Administration

CHAPTER CONTENTS

CHAPTER OBJECTIVES

Administration of Creams, Lotions, and Ointments

1. Describe the topical forms of medications used on the skin.
2. Cite the equipment needed and techniques used to apply each of the topical forms of medications to the skin surface.

Patch Testing for Allergens

1. Describe the purpose of and the procedure used for performing patch testing.
2. Describe specific charting methods used with allergy testing.

Administration of Nitroglycerin Ointment

1. Identify the equipment needed, sites used, techniques used, and patient education required when nitroglycerin ointment is prescribed.
2. Describe specific documentation methods used to record the therapeutic effectiveness of nitroglycerin ointment therapy.

Administration of Transdermal Drug Delivery Systems

1. Identify the equipment needed, sites used, techniques used, and patient education required when transdermal medication systems are prescribed.
2. Describe specific documentation methods used to record the therapeutic effectiveness of medications administered using a transdermal delivery system.

Administration of Topical Powders

1. Describe the dosage form, sites used, and techniques employed to administer medications in topical powder form.

Administration of Medications to Mucous Membranes

1. Describe the dosage forms, sites used, equipment used, and techniques employed for administration of medications to the mucous membranes.
2. Identify the dosage forms safe for administration to the eye.
3. Describe patient education necessary for patients requiring ophthalmic medications.
4. Compare the techniques used to administer eardrops in a child under three years of age and in patients over three years old.
5. Describe the purpose, precautions, and patient education for persons requiring medications by inhalation.
6. Describe the dosage forms available for vaginal administration of medications.
7. Identify the equipment needed, sites used, and specific techniques required to administer vaginal medications or douches.
8. State the rationale and procedure used for cleansing vaginal applicators or douche tips following use.
9. Develop a plan for patient education of persons taking medications via the percutaneous routes.

KEY WORDS

creams	buccal
lotions	sublingual
ointments	ophthalmic
wet dressings	otic
patch testing	nebulae
antigen	aerosols
allergen	metered dose inhalers
transdermal patch	

Copyright © 2001 by Mosby, Inc.   All rights reserved.

ASSIGNMENTS

Read textbook, pages 139-155.
Study Key Words associated with the chapter content.
Complete Chapter 10 Practice Quiz.
Complete Chapter 10 Exam.

 Copyright © 2001 by Mosby, Inc.   All rights reserved.

Review Sheet

Percutaneous Administration

Questions

1. What factors affect the absorption of topical medications?
2. What is the major advantage of the percutaneous route for drug administration?

3. Explain the differences between a cream, lotion, ointment, and wet dressing and cite the methods used to apply each.
4. What health teaching should be given a patient using a topical form of medication?
5. What is the purpose of patch testing?

6. Describe the method used to apply allergens and read results.
7. List commonly used symbols for reading of reactions to allergen testing.
8. Describe the specific method used to apply nitroglycerin ointment and a nitroglycerin transdermal disk.

9. Why is it important for the nurse to wear gloves when applying a topical ointment or transdermal patch?
10. What types of medications are available in transdermal patch form?

Answer

1. Factors affecting the absorption of topical medications include drug concentration, length of time medication is in contact with the skin, size and depth of affected area, and thickness and hydration of the skin.
2. The action of the drug is primarily limited to the site of application, thereby decreasing the systemic side effects.
3. See textbook, p. 139.

4. Patients receiving topical medications should receive the following health teaching: personal hygiene measures to treat/improve underlying condition, methods of application, ways to avoid touching affected areas, and prevention of spread of infection when present.
5. Patch testing is used to identify specific sensitivity to allergens.
6. See textbook, pp. 141-143.

7. Commonly used symbols for reading allergen patch test reactions include (see also p. 142):

+	1+ erythema
++	2+ erythema and papules
+++	3+ erythema, papules and vesicles
++++	4+ generalized fusing of blistered areas

8. See textbook, pp. 143-144.

9. The nurse should wear gloves when administering a topical ointment or transdermal patch to avoid inadvertent absorption of the medication by the nurse through the skin.

11. Why is it important to discard transdermal medication patches safely after removal?

12. Where are sublingual and buccal forms of medication administered?

13. What is the primary advantage of the sublingual route?

14. What abbreviations are used for ophthalmic medications?

15. Describe the correct techniques for administering eye drops and eye ointments, including patient teaching.

16. Compare the correct technique of administering an ear (otic) drug to a child and to an adult.

17. Explain the procedure for instilling nose drops/nasal sprays into an adult and a child; include health teaching.

18. Why shouldn't oily preparations be administered by inhalation?

19. Explain how to give medications by inhalation.

20. What is a metered dose inhaler?

21. Explain how to teach a patient to administer a medication using an inhaler.

22. Explain the correct technique for inserting a vaginal suppository and proper hygiene measures used during the course of treatment.

10. Nitroglycerin, clonidine, estrogen, nicotine, scopolamine, and fentanyl are available in transdermal patch forms.

11. Used transdermal patches must be safely discarded because the patch may still contain some medication which could be harmful to individuals or pets for whom it is not prescribed.

12. Sublingual medications are administered under the tongue; buccal medications are administered in the back cheek area of the mouth.

13. In addition to being easy to access, the sublingual area provides rapid absorption and onset of action of the drug because the drug passes directly into the systemic circulation with no immediate pass-through the liver, where extensive metabolism usually takes place.

14. All medications used in the eye should be specifically labeled FOR OPHTHALMIC USE. Abbreviations used are:
os = left eye
od = right eye
ou = both eyes

15. See textbook, pp. 147-149.

16. See textbook, pp. 149-150.

17. See textbook, pp. 150-151.

18. Oily preparations should not be administered by inhaler because oil droplets would be carried to the lungs and initiate a lipid pneumonia.

19. See textbook, pp. 152-153.

20. A metered dose inhaler is an aerosolized, pressurized inhaler that delivers a measured amount of medication with each depression of the device.

21. See textbook, p. 153.

22. See textbook, pp. 153-154.

Copyright © 2001 by Mosby, Inc. All rights reserved.

CHAPTER 10

Practice Quiz

Percutaneous Administration

ESSAY

1. When applying topical drugs, the site should be cleansed prior to application of the new dose of medication. Explain how to cleanse the site correctly.
2. Why are gloves worn when applying topical dosage forms of medication?
3. Which type of topical medication needs to be shaken well prior to administration?
4. Describe the correct techniques for application of ointments and creams.

CHARTING

Chart the essential data in the following situation.

M.T. has a red, weeping, ulcerated area on the lower leg that is to be dressed using neomycin powder. Use today's date and time when doing the charting.

MEDICATION ADMINISTRATION RECORD

NAME:		RM-BD:		Init	Signature	Title
ID NO.:		AGE:				
DIAGNOSIS:		SEX:				

PHYSICIAN:		Ht:		Wt:	

SCHEDULED MEDICATIONS

DATE	MEDICATION-STRENGTH-FORM-ROUTE	0030-0729	0730-1529	1530-0029

** PRN MEDICATIONS**

Copyright © 2001 by Mosby, Inc.   All rights reserved.

5. M.T. is to receive 1/2" of nitroglycerin topical ointment at 9 P.M. Explain how to measure and apply the dose at site 8 on the figure below. Chart the medication using today's date on M.T.'s chart in the situation above.

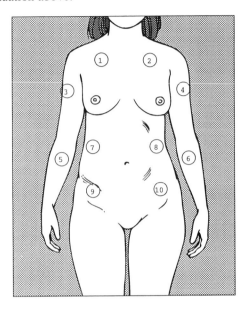

6. Explain the correct technique for applying a topical disk containing nitroglycerin and state the patient teaching that would be appropriate while performing this task.

7. A.H. is using nitroglycerin sublingually and is keeping the medication at the bedside. What data would you collect during and at the end of the shift to include in the charting?

8. Use M.T.'s chart already provided to chart the following medication:
    Timoptic one drop in both eyes at 8 A.M. daily

9. Describe the correct technique for instilling eye drops.

10. Explain the rationale for blocking the inner corner (canthus) of the eye for 1-2 minutes after instilling an eye medication.

11. Differentiate between the direction you pull the earlobe in a child under three years old and in an adult when instilling ear drops.

12. Why should you have the individual blow his/her nose gently prior to instilling nose drops or a nasal spray?

13. Describe the health teaching that should be completed when nasal spray or nose drops are being used.

14. Explain the procedure for administering a medication using a metered-dose inhaler.

15. Explain the procedure for positioning the patient, inserting the medication, and providing follow-up care to a patient having a vaginal cream inserted.

Copyright © 2001 by Mosby, Inc. All rights reserved.

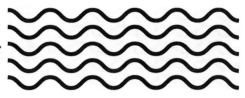

CHAPTER 11

Syllabus

Drugs Affecting the Autonomic Nervous System

CHAPTER CONTENTS

CHAPTER OBJECTIVES

1. Differentiate between afferent and efferent nerve conduction within the central nervous system.
2. Explain the role of neurotransmitters at synaptic junctions.
3. Name the most common neurotransmitters known to affect central nervous system function.
4. Identify the two major neurotransmitters of the autonomic nervous system.
5. Cite the names of nerve endings liberating acetylcholine and those liberating norepinephrine.
6. Explain the action of drugs that inhibit the actions of cholinergic and adrenergic fibers.
7. Identify two broad classes of drugs used to stimulate the adrenergic nervous system.
8. Name the neurotransmitters called catecholamines.
9. Review the actions of adrenergic agents to identify conditions that would be affected favorably and unfavorably by these medications.
10. Explain the rationale for using adrenergic blocking agents for conditions that have vasoconstriction as part of the disease pathophysiology.
11. Describe the benefits of using beta-adrenergic blocking agents for hypertension, angina pectoris, cardiac arrhythmias, and hyperthyroidism.
12. Identify disease conditions that would preclude the use of beta-adrenergic blocking agents.
13. List the neurotransmitters responsible for cholinergic activity.
14. List the predictable side effects of cholinergic agents.
15. List the predictable side effects anticholinergic agents.
16. Describe the clinical uses of anticholinergic agents.

KEY WORDS

central nervous system
afferent nerves
efferent nerves
peripheral nervous system
motor nervous system
autonomic nervous system
neurons
synapse
neurotransmitters
norepinephrine

acetylcholine
cholinergic fibers
adrenergic fibers
anticholinergic agent
adrenergic blocking agent
catecholamine
alpha receptor
beta receptor
dopaminergic receptors

ASSIGNMENTS

Read textbook, pp. 158-167.
Study Key Words associated with the chapter content.
Study Review Sheet for Chapter 11.
Complete Practice Quiz for Chapter 11.
Complete Chapter 11 Exam.

Copyright © 2001 by Mosby, Inc.   All rights reserved.

CHAPTER

11

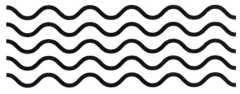

Review Sheet

Drugs Affecting the Autonomic Nervous System

The QUESTION column and the ANSWER column have been offset so that you can cover the answer while reading the question, allowing you to assess your knowledge.

Question

1. The central nervous system is composed of _____.
2. The autonomic nervous system relays information from the central nervous system to _____.
3. The autonomic nervous system controls the functions of what types of tissue?

4. What primary function is controlled by the motor nervous system?
5. What neurotransmitter is liberated by cholinergic fibers?
6. What neurotransmitter is liberated by adrenergic fibers?
7. What three major types of receptors are found in the autonomic nervous system?
8. Stimulation of alpha$_1$ receptors causes what action on blood vessels?

9. Stimulation of beta$_1$ receptors produces what type of effect on the heart rate?

10. Stimulation of beta$_2$ receptors produces what effects?

11. Define *adrenergic agent*.

12. When beta adrenergic agents are administered, what effects will be seen on blood vessels, bronchi, heart rate, blood pressure, respiration, lungs, gastric motility and tone, and blood glucose?

Answer

1. The central nervous system is composed of the brain and spinal cord.
2. The autonomic nervous system relays information from the central nervous system (CNS) to the whole body.
3. The autonomic nervous system controls the functions of all tissue except striated muscle.
4. Skeletal muscle contractions are controlled by the motor nervous system.
5. The cholinergic fibers secrete acetylcholine.

6. The adrenergic fibers secrete norepinephrine.

7. The three major types of receptors found in the autonomic nervous system (ANS) are "alpha," "beta," and "dopaminergic" receptors.
8. Stimulation of alpha$_1$ receptors causes vasoconstriction. This results in a rise in blood pressure; therefore, before giving alpha$_1$-type medications, the blood pressure should be checked. This action makes these drugs useful in the treatment of hypotension and shock.
9. Stimulation of beta$_1$ receptors increases the heart rate. If excessive doses of a beta$_1$ agonist are administered, the patient may experience tachycardia and arrhythmias.
10. Stimulation of beta$_2$ receptors relaxes the smooth muscle of the bronchi, uterus, and peripheral blood vessels. These actions make these drugs useful as bronchodilators and inhibitors of preterm labor.
11. An adrenergic agent produces or mimics the effects of stimulation of the sympathetic nervous system. Therefore, these drugs are also known as "sympathomimetic" agents.

Copyright © 2001 by Mosby, Inc.   All rights reserved.

13. What premedication assessments should be completed prior to administering an adrenergic agent?

14. Giving an excessive dose of an adrenergic agent results in what adverse effects?

15. List the primary actions of alpha-adrenergic blocking agents and beta-adrenergic blocking agents.

16. Why/when are alpha- and beta-adrenergic blocking agents prescribed?

17. State the possible effects of administering beta blockers to a patient with a known respiratory disease such as asthma or emphysema.

18. Which portion of the autonomic nervous system do cholinergic agents affect?

19. What effect do beta blockers have on a patient with diabetes mellitus?

20. What pharmacologic effect may be expected when indomethacin and beta blocker therapy are combined?

21. What drug is a specific antidote for cholinergic agents?

22. Under what types of clinical conditions are cholinergic agents be used?

23. What side effects can be anticipated when an anticholinergic agent is administered?

24. What actions of anticholinergic agents make them useful in the clinical treatment of gastrointestinal disorders?

12. When adrenergic agents are administered, blood vessels dilate, bronchi dilate, heart rate increases, blood pressure may drop, GI peristalsis decreases, relaxation of the gastric smooth muscle occurs, and blood glucose increases.

13. Before administering an adrenergic agent, the following assessments should be completed: baseline vital signs (e.g., heart rate, blood pressure), screen for respiratory tract disease, and ascertain if the patients uses bronchodilators or decongestants.

14. Excessive doses of an adrenergic agent may result in arrhythmias, hypertension, nervousness, anxiety, and insomnia due to stimulation of the sympathetic nervous system.

15. Alpha-adrenergic blocking agents act by plugging the alpha receptors, preventing vasoconstriction of arterioles. Beta-adrenergic blocking agents act by plugging the beta-adrenergic receptors, preventing beta stimulation, especially from norepinephrine and epinephrine.

16. Alpha-adrenergic blocking agents are used to treat diseases with vasoconstriction (e.g., peripheral vascular disease, Buerger's disease, and Raynaud's disease). Beta blocking agents are used to treat hypertension, angina pectoris, cardiac arrhythmias, and hyperthyroidism.

17. Administering a beta blocker to a person with a known respiratory disease may cause broncho-constriction and make the person experience respiratory distress.

18. Cholinergic agents affect the parasympathetic portion of the nervous system.

19. Beta blockers induce hypoglycemia; they decrease the release of insulin in response to hypoglycemia and mask the symptoms normally associated with hypoglycemia.

20. The combination of indomethacin and beta blocker therapy may cause loss of hypertensive control. The dosage of the beta blocker may need to be increased.

21. Atropine sulfate, an anticholinergic agent, is a specific antidote for cholinergic agents.

22. Cholinergic agents can be used to treat glaucoma, urinary retention, myasthenia gravis, as a muscle relaxant to reverse nondepolarizing agents, and for gastrointestinal disorders such as paralytic ileus.

23. Anticholinergic agents produce the following side effects: dryness of mouth and tongue, blurring of vision, mild nausea, and nervousness. Other side effects include constipation, urinary hesitancy or retention, tachycardia, palpitations, mydriasis, muscle cramping, and mild transient postural hypotension.

Copyright © 2001 by Mosby, Inc. All rights reserved.

25. Before administering any anticholinergic agent, the patient's history should be checked for the presence of what type of eye disorder?

26. Atropine is an example of an anticholinergic agent frequently used preoperatively. Which of the drug's anticholinergic properties make this drug useful preoperatively?

27. What premedication assessments should be completed before administering an anticholinergic agent?

28. What side effects can be anticipated whenever an anticholinergic agent is administered?

29. The postoperative patient who has been given atropine sulfate needs to be monitored for

_____.

30. Describe the action(s) and side effects of the following drug classifications and/or drugs: alpha adrenergic agents, beta adrenergic agents, cholinergic agents, anticholinergic agents, beta adrenergic blocking agents, physostigmine, epinephrine, and atropine.

24. Anticholinergic (also known as antispasmodic) agents' actions include decreased secretion of saliva, hydrochloric acid, pepsin, bile, and other enzymatic fluids necessary for digestion, along with relaxation of the sphincter muscles and decreased spasm, which allows peristalsis to move the contents of the stomach and bowel through the gastrointestinal tract.

25. All patients' charts should be screened for the presence of angle-closure glaucoma before any anticholinergic agent is administered.

26. Atropine sulfate is given preoperatively to dry secretions of the mouth, nose, throat, and bronchi, and decrease secretions during surgery. It also prevents vagal stimulation and bradycardia during the placement of the endotracheal tube.

27. Check for a history of angle-closure glaucoma or history of enlarged prostate and urinary hesitancy or retention before administering an anticholinergic agent.

28. Anticholinergic agents produce the following side effects: dry mouth and tongue, blurred vision, mild nausea, and nervousness. Other side effects include constipation, urinary hesitancy or retention, tachycardia, palpitations, mydriasis, muscle cramping, and mild transient postural hypotension.

29. The postoperative patient who received atropine sulfate needs to be monitored frequently for urinary retention. There may also be postoperative constipation.

30. See textbook, pp. 159-167. Examine drug monographs and drug classification explanations.

Copyright © 2001 by Mosby, Inc.   All rights reserved.

 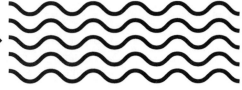

Practice Quiz

Drugs Affecting the Autonomic Nervous System

COMPLETION

Complete the following statements.

1. Catecholamines that are secreted naturally in the body are _____, _____, and _____.
2. Dopamine is secreted at what three primary sites in the body? _____, _____, _____.
3. The three types of sympathetic autonomic nervous system receptors are _____, _____, and _____.
4. Cholinergic agents are also known as _____.
5. Stimulation of the adrenergic receptors causes _____ of the bronchial muscles, which causes _____ of the airway.
6. Stimulation of the cholinergic receptors causes _____ of bronchial muscles, which causes _____ of the airway.
7. Prior to administration of an adrenergic agent, what premedication assessments should be done?
8. List two common side effects to expect with the administration of adrenergic agents.
9. When an anticholinergic agent is prescribed what monitoring should be done?
10. The generic names of all beta$_1$ blocking agents end in "-____".

Describe the action(s) of the following agents.

11. Cholinergics _____.
12. Beta adrenergics _____.
13. Alpha adrenergics _____.
14. Beta-adrenergic blockers _____.

ESSAY

1. Based on a review of this chapter, related to the actions, uses, and side effects of the primary drug classifications (adrenergic, adrenergic blocking agents, cholinergic, anticholinergic agents), develop a list of premedication assessments that should be made before using these drugs.
2. Summarize the actions of the cholinergic and anticholinergic agents. Arrange the summaries in columns to compare cholinergic and anticholinergic actions.
3. Examine the drug actions listed for adrenergic blocking agents. Explain the mechanisms by which these drugs are beneficial for the treatment of angina pectoris, cardiac arrhythmias, and hypertension.
4. Explain the effect of vasoconstriction and vasodilation of blood vessels on blood pressure.
5. What type of autonomic system drugs should not be used in persons with pulmonary disorders?

END-OF-CHAPTER MATH REVIEW

1. Order: Benadryl 40 mg po, tid. Benadryl 12.5 mg/5 ml is available. Give: _____.
2. Order: Propranolol 60 mg po, tid. Propranolol 40 mg tablets is available. Give: _____.
3. Ordered: Atropine sulfate gr 1/150 sc preoperatively "on call." Atropine sulfate 0.3, 0.4, and 0.5 mg/ml is available. Give: _____.

Copyright © 2001 by Mosby, Inc.   All rights reserved.

CHAPTER 12

Sedative-Hypnotics

Syllabus

CHAPTER CONTENTS

CHAPTER OBJECTIVES

1. Differentiate among the terms *sedative* and *hypnotic; initial, intermittent,* and *terminal insomnia;* and *rebound sleep* and *paradoxic excitement.*
2. Identify alterations found in the sleep pattern when hypnotics are discontinued.
3. Cite nursing interventions that can be implemented as alternatives to administering a sedative/hypnotic.
4. Compare the effects of barbiturates and benzodiazepines on the central nervous system.
5. Explain the major benefits of administering benzodiazepines rather than barbiturates.
6. Identify laboratory tests that should be monitored when benzodiazepines or barbiturates are administered over an extended period.
7. Develop a patient education plan for a patient receiving a hypnotic.

KEY WORDS

paradoxic sleep
REM sleep
insomnia
hypnotic
sedative
rebound sleep

ASSIGNMENTS

Read textbook, pp. 168-177.
Study Key Words associated with chapter content.
Study Review Sheet for Chapter 12.
Complete End-of-Chapter Math Review and Critical Thinking Questions.
Assign Collaborative Activity as appropriate.
Complete Chapter 12 Practice Quiz.
Complete Chapter 12 Exam.

COLLABORATIVE ACTIVITIES

Complete the following activities to prepare for in-class discussion and group work that may be assigned by the instructor.

1. Perform an interview. Use information in "Nursing Process for Sedative-Hypnotics" to formulate a data assessment, develop questions, and interview a family member, neighbor, or friend who has complained about inability to sleep.
2. Read two articles on sleep disturbance or on the drug classes of the benzodiazepines or barbiturates and bring a copy of the article to a conference. Be prepared to summarize the article and discuss how it applies to the topic being studied.
3. During the post-interview conference, answer the following questions:
   a. What type of sleep pattern disturbance is present?
   b. Is anxiety contributing to the problem?
   c. What type of sleeping environment is present?
   d. Does the individual use caffeine?
4. After examining the data collected, discuss possible interventions to help alleviate the problem without drugs.

(Note to student: Attend a follow-up conference with your instructor to discuss data or to seek guidance with this project.)

Copyright © 2001 by Mosby, Inc.   All rights reserved.

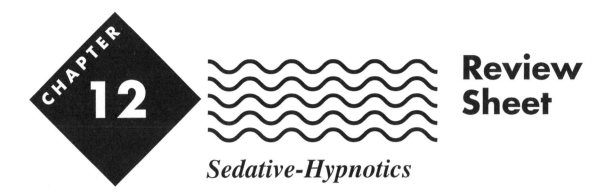

Review Sheet

Sedative-Hypnotics

The QUESTION column and the ANSWER column have been offset so that you can cover the answer while reading the questions, allowing you to assess your knowledge.

Question	Answer
1. What are the four stages of sleep?	1. Sleep stages I-IV are explained in textbook, p. 168.
2. What is another name for paradoxic sleep?	
3. What is insomnia?	2. Rapid eye movement (REM) sleep is also called paradoxic sleep.
	3. Insomnia is the inability to sleep.
4. What premedication assessments should be performed prior to administering any sedative/hypnotic agent?	
5. Differentiate between the actions of a sedative and a hypnotic.	4. Before administering a sedative/hypnotic agent, assess for level of alertness, orientation, and ability to perform motor functions, as well as current blood pressure, pulse, respirations, sleep pattern, anxiety level, and environmental and nutritional factors that might impede sleep.
6. What should a nursing history relating to a patient's complaints of insomnia include?	5. Hypnotics produce sleep. Sedatives relax the patient.
7. Name two classes of drugs used as sedative/hypnotics. What ending appears on the generic drug names?	6. A nursing history related ot a patient's complaints of insomnia should include usual pattern of sleep, anxiety level, environmental factors, nutritional habit, and medications or actions tried before seeking current treatment.
8. State the effect of hypnotics on respiratory function.	7. Two classes of sedative/hypnotics are barbiturates (all end in "-tal") and benzodiazepines (all end in "-am", except chlordiazepoxide [Librium]).
	8. Hypnotics produce mild to marked respiratory depression, depending on dosage and pulmonary function.
9. What changes in REM sleep occur with the administration of barbiturates?	9. Barbiturates produce initially decreased REM sleep; however, as tolerance builds, REM sleep returns to normal.
10. What is a rebound effect associated with discontinuing barbiturates?	
11. What is meant by morning hangover associated with barbiturates, benzodiazepines, and miscellaneous agents used as sedative/hypnotics? State the associated health teaching that needs to be initiated.	10. A rebound effect associated with discontinuing barbiturates is increase in REM; it may take several weeks following barbiturate therapy for this to resolve.

Copyright © 2001 by Mosby, Inc.   All rights reserved.

12. What is a paradoxical response to hypnotics and what nursing actions are required if this response occurs?

13. What laboratory studies are recommended with continued use of barbiturates and benzodiazepines?

14. List the generic and brand names of commonly prescribed barbiturates, benzodiazepines, and miscellaneous sedative/hypnotic agents as assigned by the instructor.

15. In addition to their use as sedative/hypnotics, for what other clinical uses are barbiturates prescribed?

16. What effect can the regular use of barbiturates have on oral contraceptive therapy?

17. What is the blood-brain barrier?

18. What side effects can be expected from the administration of sedative/hypnotics?

19. What are side effects to report when taking sedative/hypnotics?

20. What premedication assessments should be performed before administration of a benzodiazepine?

11. Morning hangover from sedative/hypnotics includes blurred vision, mental dullness, and mild hypotension. Health teaching about this effect should include directions to consult M.D. if these symptoms become too bothersome; instructions to rise slowly to sitting position, equilibrate, then stand; and a caution regarding use of machinery, etc.

12. Paradoxical response is a period of excitement prior to sedation induced by use of barbiturates and other sedative/hypnotics not usually associated with benzodiazepine therapy. Appropriate nursing actions include protecting patient from harm providing for channeling of energy.

13. RBC, WBC, and differential count lab studies should be done with continued use of barbiturates and benzodiazepines. Also report immediately sore throat, fever, progressive weakness, purpura, or jaundice.

14. Consult Tables 12-1, p. 172; 12-2, p. 174; and 12-3, p. 176.

15. Specific agents are used as anticonvulsants and induction anesthetics.

16. The client may need to use an alternative form of contraceptive therapy, particularly if spotting or breakthrough bleeding occurs.

17. The blood-brain barrier is a membrane that controls the passage of drugs into the central nervous system to the receptor sites on the cells within the central nervous system.

18. Side effects of sedative/hypnotics include hangover, sedation, lethargy, blurred vision, and transient hypotension.

19. Side effects to report of sedative/hypnotics are excessive use or abuse, paradoxical response, pruritus, rash, high fever, sore throat, purpura, and jaundice.

20. Before administering a benzodiazepine, assess vital signs, including blood pressure in lying and sitting positions. Check whether the client is in the first trimester of pregnancy, breast-feeding, or has a history of a blood dyscrasia or hepatic disease.

Copyright © 2001 by Mosby, Inc. All rights reserved.

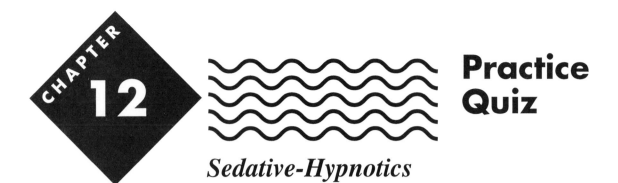

CHAPTER 12

Practice Quiz

Sedative-Hypnotics

COMPLETION

Use the following vocabulary words to complete the statements: sedative, hypnotic, rebound sleep, paradoxic excitement, initial insomnia, intermittent insomnia, terminal insomnia.

S.C. has difficulty falling asleep and the physician he consults tells him this is (1) _____ insomnia. While at the sleep disorder clinic, S.C. tells another patient, W.S., about his difficulty sleeping. W.S. quickly explains this isn't the same as his problem. He falls asleep, but awakens about 4 A.M. and can't get back to sleep. W.S.'s insomnia pattern is called (2) _____ insomnia.

Prior to surgery, the physician prescribes a(n) (3) _____ to help J.T. to sleep the night prior to surgery. The next morning, a (4) _____ is ordered for 8 A.M. (0800) for the purpose of providing relaxation and rest while awaiting scheduled surgery at 10:30 A.M. (1030). Two days after surgery, J.T. asks the nurse if it would be okay to ask the doctor for a prescription for the "wonderful medication" she took prior to surgery because she had the best sleep that day. The nurse asked her about her sleep pattern. She described that she generally has difficulty sleeping all night at home. She sleeps awhile, awakens, and sleeps in cycles several times nightly. The nurse tells her this is known as (5) _____ insomnia.

Develop a response to J.T.'s question regarding her intention to request a prescription for a (6) _____ from the physician for use at home. Include in the explanation why long-term use of sedative-hypnotics is not beneficial and explain rebound sleep in lay terms.

Based on the data given for J.T.'s situation, develop two nursing diagnosis statements appropriate for her case.

7. _____

8. _____

9. List the side effects that can be anticipated with the administration of barbiturates and benzodiazepines.

Barbiturates: _____

Benzodiazepines: _____

10. What is meant by the statement that a drug produces physical dependence?

11. What premedication assessments should be performed prior to the administration of ANY sedative/hypnotic? Which assessments should be completed prior to administering a benzodiazepine or a barbiturate?

ESSAY

1. Three hours after being given a hypnotic, C.G. is still awake. She is having major surgery in the morning. Describe the actions you should initiate and the rationale for performing each.
2. Why should patients be cautioned against the use of alcohol when taking sedative/hypnotics?
3. Describe situations in which repeating a dose of a sedative/hypnotic would be appropriate.

END-OF-CHAPTER MATH REVIEW

1. Dr. Smith wrote orders to start J.H. on triazolam 0.5 mg at bedtime 4 days only. Triazolam is available in 0.125 and 0.25 mg tablets. What will you administer?
2. Dr. Jones wrote orders for J.S. to receive 400 mg of chloral hydrate 1 hour before a computed tomography scan. Chloral hydrate is available in 250 and 500 mg capsules and 250 and 500 mg/5 ml syrup. What will you administer?
3. L.H. is scheduled for an endoscopy at 9 A.M. tomorrow morning. He weighs 60 kg. A dose of midazolam 7.5 mg IV is scheduled to be administered a few minutes before the endoscopy. The normal midazolam dose is 0.1 to 0.15 mg/kg. Is the 7.5 mg dose a reasonable dose for this patient?

      Copyright © 2001 by Mosby, Inc.   All rights reserved.

Syllabus

Drugs Used for Parkinson's Disease

CHAPTER CONTENT

Parkinson's Disease (p. 178)
> Drug Therapy for Treatment of Parkinson's Disease
> > (p. 179)
> Drug Class: Dopamine Agonists (p. 182)
> Drug Class: COMT Inhibitor (p. 188)
> Drug Class: Anticholinergic Agents (p. 189)
> Drug Class: Miscellaneous Antiparkinson's Agents
> > (p. 190)

CHAPTER OBJECTIVES

1. List signs and symptoms of Parkinson's disease and accurately define the vocabulary used for the pharmacologic agents prescribed and the disease state.
2. Name the neurotransmitter that is found in excess and the neurotransmitter that is deficient in persons with parkinsonism.
3. Describe reasonable expectations of medications prescribed for treatment of Parkinson's disease.
4. Identify the period of time necessary for a therapeutic response to be observed when drug therapy for parkinsonism is initiated.
5. Name the action of bromocriptine mesylate, carbidopa, levodopa, and tolcapone neurotransmitters involved in Parkinson's disease.
6. List symptoms that can be attributed to the cholinergic activity of pharmacologic agents.
7. Name the actions of bromocriptine mesylate, carbidopa, and levodopa on neurotransmitters involved in Parkinson's disease.
8. Cite the specific symptoms that should show improvement when anticholinergic agents are administered to the patient with Parkinson's disease.
9. Develop a health teaching plan for an individual being treated with levodopa.

KEY WORDS

Parkinson's disease
dopamine
neurotransmitter
acetylcholine
tremor

dyskinesia
propulsive movements
livedo reticularis
anticholinergic agents

ASSIGNMENTS

Read textbook, pp. 179-191.
Study Key Words associated with the chapter content.
Study Review Sheet for Chapter 13.
Complete End-of-Chapter Math Review and Critical
> Thinking Questions.
Assign Collaborative Activity as appropriate.
Complete Chapter 13 Practice Quiz.
Complete Chapter 13 Exam.

COLLABORATIVE ACTIVITIES

Complete the following activities. Be prepared to share your responses during in-class discussion or group work that may be assigned by the instructor.
1. Select a patient with Parkinson's disease.
2. What medications, of those listed on the MAR (medication administration record), are specifically used to treat this disease?
3. List the desired action of each antiparkinsonian medication prescribed.
4. Develop focused assessments that can be used to detect a positive or negative response to these drugs.
5. Discuss the findings in class, conference, or a seminar setting.

Copyright © 2001 by Mosby, Inc.   All rights reserved.

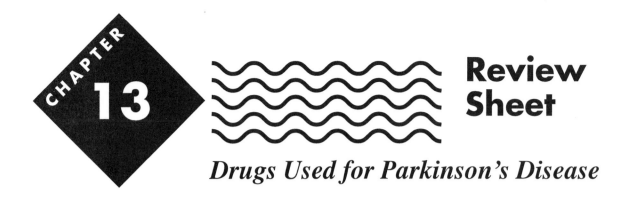

Review Sheet

Drugs Used for Parkinson's Disease

The QUESTION column and the ANSWER column have been offset so that you can cover the answer while reading the question, allowing you to assess your knowledge.

Question	Answer
1. Prepare a list of signs and symptoms of parkinsonism.	
2. Summarize the purpose of giving medications to treat Parkinson's disease.	1. Signs and symptoms of parkinsonism are expressionlessness; mask-like face; tremors of hands, lips, tongue, and jaw; "pill-rolling" movements of fingers; excessive salivation; and dyskinesia.
3. Identify the basic components of a baseline assessment of a patient's neurologic function.	2. Medications are given to treat Parkinson's disease to provide maximum relief of symptoms and to optimize independence of movement and activity.
4. Persons taking amantadine hydrochloride may experience confusion, disorientation, and mental depression. What actions should the nurse take if/when this occurs?	3. Baseline neurologic assessment includes orientation to name, date, time, and place; degree of alertness; ability to comprehend and follow instructions; and degree of involvement in daily activities of self.
5. Because of the many side effects known to occur with medications used to treat parkinsonism, what health teaching should be initiated?	4. The nurse should provide for patient safety, report alterations for evaluation by the physician, and continue to make regularly scheduled assessments of the individual's neurologic status.
6. Compare the actions of amantadine hydrochloride, bromocriptine mesylate, carbidopa, levodopa, pergolide mesylate, selegiline, and tolcapone.	5. Prepare a list of symptoms the patient has before starting therapy and involve the patient in keeping track of alterations (as the individual's abilities permit). Explain the need for continuing therapy for a period sufficient for the effectiveness of medications to be evaluated. Have patient report effects that are particularly bothersome; work cooperatively to plan approaches to alleviate the problems.
7. Summarize the side effects associated with medication therapy used in the treatment of parkinsonism. State nursing actions that could be used to alleviate and/or prevent the side effects.	6. Amantadine hydrochloride slows destruction of dopamine and may aid in release of dopamine from storage sites. Bromocriptine mesylate stimulates dopamine receptors in basal ganglia of the brain. Carbidopa inhibits the metabolism of levodopa. Levodopa replaces dopamine deficiency in the basal ganglia of the brain. Pergolide mesylate stimulates postsynaptic dopamine receptors. Selegiline has an unknown mechanism of action. Tolcapone reduces the destruction of dopamine in peripheral tissue allowing significantly more to reach the brain.

Copyright © 2001 by Mosby, Inc.   All rights reserved.

8. What type of glaucoma prohibits the use of levodopa?

9. What specific type of vitamin preparation should be used by patients taking levodopa?

10. list three drugs used to treat parkinsonism.

11. What drug may be combined with levodopa to improve its effectiveness?

12. Persons taking levodopa (Larodopa) for several months may develop what type of central nervous system side effects?

13. Why should a baseline neurologic assessment be done prior to and periodically during the administration of commonly prescribed drugs for treatment of Parkinson's disease?

14. What neurologic side effects are most often seen with pergolide?

15. What is the primary mechanism of action of anticholinergic agents?

16. What are the therapeutic outcomes desired when an anticholinergic agent is prescribed for a Parkinson's patient?

17. When the ability to perform motor functions is impaired, what nursing diagnosis statement could be made?

7. See p. 183 (amantadine), p. 184 (bromocriptine), p. 185 (levodopa), p. 186 (pergolide), p. 188 (tolcapone), and p. 189 (anticholinergic agents).

8. Angle-closure glaucoma prohibits the use of levodopa.

9. Pyridoxine-free multiple vitamin (Larobec) should be used by patients taking levodopa.

10. Drugs used to treat parkinsonism include bromocriptine mesylate (Parlodel), levodopa (Larodopa), amantadine (Symmetrel), carbidopa (Sinemet), and pergolide mesylate (Permax).

11. Carbidopa, an enzyme inhibitor that reduces the metabolism of levodopa, allows a greater portion of the administered levodopa to reach the receptor sites in the basal ganglia.

12. Long-term use of levodopa can cause abnormal movements (e.g., rocking, facial grimacing, chewing motions, head and neck bobbing).

13. Several of the drugs use to treat Parkinson's disease can cause adverse effects such as confusion and hallucinations. It is important to know which is a progression of the disease and which is due to an adverse effect of drug therapy.

14. Common neurologic side effects with pergolide include dyskinesia, hallucinations, somnolence, and insomnia.

15. The primary mechanism of action of anticholinergic agents is to reduce overstimulation caused by the excess of acetylcholine, a cholinergic neurotransmitter.

16. The desired effects are reduction in drooling, sweating, tremors, and depression.

17. Injury, Risk for, related to Parkinson's disease; manifested by propulsive gait, unsteadiness, and progressive inability to walk unassisted

Copyright © 2001 by Mosby, Inc. All rights reserved.

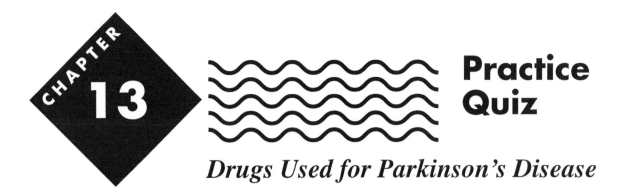

CHAPTER 13

Practice Quiz

Drugs Used for Parkinson's Disease

COMPLETION

Complete the following statements.

1. With Parkinson's disease, the neurotransmitter _____ is deficient, leaving a relative excess of the neurotransmitter _____.

2. The primary goals of drug therapy for the treatment of Parkinson's disease are _____ and _____.

3. List five symptoms of Parkinson's disease.

4. State two nursing diagnoses that may occur when medicines are administered to treat Parkinson's disease (for example, levodopa-carbidopa, bromocriptine mesylate).

5. When a drug monograph lists orthostatic hypotension as a possible adverse effect, what nursing actions should be implemented?

6. How is a person's mental status assessed?

7. How soon after initiation of drug therapy for Parkinson's disease will a therapeutic response be seen?

8. To help reduce an excess amount of acetylcholine, _____ agents are prescribed.

9. All patients receiving levodopa should have the following premedication assessment:

10. The major action of the drug carbidopa is:

11. The major action of the drug levodopa is:

12. The major action of the drug tolcapone is:

ESSAY

1. What physiologic effect does stimulation of dopamine receptors have?

2. G.H.'s family asks you to explain the basic underlying problem that is causing the symptoms of Parkinson's disease in their mother. Give a simple explanation of the symptoms, appropriate for use with a lay person. Include an explanation of neurotransmitters and the basic imbalances found with Parkinson's disease.

3. Discuss the normal course of progression of Parkinson's disease and include the rationale for drug therapy to alleviate the symptoms.

4. Develop a teaching plan to be used with the patient and family of an individual being started on Sinemet for the treatment of Parkinson's disease.

5. Explain baseline assessment of an individual's mental status and physical symptoms that are important before and periodically throughout the course of treatment of Parkinson's disease.

6. F.J. is being started on an anticholinergic drug as part of the treatment plan for Parkinson's disease. What symptoms could you anticipate improvement in and conversely, what problems could also arise from starting this medication?

END-OF-CHAPTER MATH REVIEW

1. Dr. Jones wrote orders to start R.L. on Sinemet 25/100 mg at an initial dose of one tablet tid. Sinemet is available in ratios of 10/100, 25/100, 25/250, and 50/200 mg strengths. Which strength should be used and how many tablets should be administered for each individual dose?

2. Dr. Jones wrote orders to start K.J. on levodopa 0.25 g qid. Levodopa is available in 100, 250, and 500 mg strengths. Which strength should be used and how many tablets should be administered at one time?

3. Dr. Jones wrote to start A.S. on bromocriptine at an initial dose of 1.25 mg 2 times daily with meals. Bromocriptine is available in 2.5 mg. tablets and 5 mg capsules. What will you administer?

Copyright © 2001 by Mosby, Inc.   All rights reserved.

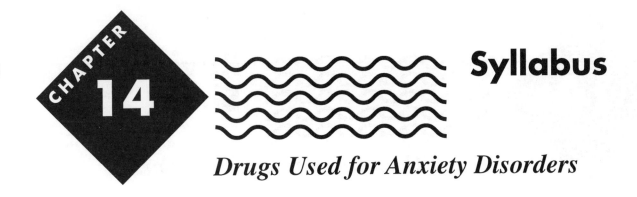

CHAPTER 14

Drugs Used for Anxiety Disorders

Syllabus

CHAPTER CONTENT

Anxiety Disorders (p. 192)
  Drug Therapy for Anxiety Disorders (p. 193)
  Drug Class: Benzodiazepines (p. 195)
  Drug Class: Azaspirones (p. 198)
  Drug Class: Selective Serotonin Reuptake Inhibitors
    (p. 198)
  Drug Class: Miscellaneous Agents (p. 198)

CHAPTER OBJECTIVES

1. Define terminology associated with anxiety states.
2. Describe the essential components of a baseline assessment of a patient's mental status.
3. Cite the side effects of hydroxyzine therapy and identify those effects requiring close monitoring when the drug is used preoperatively.
4. Develop a teaching plan for patient education of persons taking antianxiety medications.
5. Describe signs and symptoms indicating a positive therapeutic outcome in a patient being treated for a high-anxiety state.
6. Discuss psychologic and physiologic drug dependence.

KEY WORDS

anxiety
panic disorder
phobias
obsession
compulsion
anxiolytics
tranquilizers

ASSIGNMENT

Read textbook, pp. 192-200.
Study Key Words associated with chapter content.
Study Review Sheet for Chapter 14.
Complete End-of-Chapter Math Review and Critical
    Thinking Questions.
Collaborative Activity, as assigned.
Complete Chapter 14 Practice Quiz.
Complete Chapter 14 Exam.

COLLABORATIVE ACTIVITIES

Answer the following questions. Be prepared to share your responses during in-class discussion and group work that may be assigned by the instructor.

1. When hydroxyzine (Vistaril, Atarax) is used preoperatively and postoperatively, what side effects can be expected and what assessments should be made to detect them? When side effects are present, what nursing actions are appropriate?
2. Explain how to prepare the following preoperative drug orders for administration:
   Hydroxyzine 50 mg, IM on call to operating room.
   Demerol 75 mg, IM on call to operating room.
3. What nursing assessments should be performed on a regular basis on a patient who has an anxiety disorder?
4. What premedication assessments should be performed before administering hydroxyzine?
5. Explain appropriate health teaching for a patient being started on meprobamate therapy.

Copyright © 2001 by Mosby, Inc.   All rights reserved.

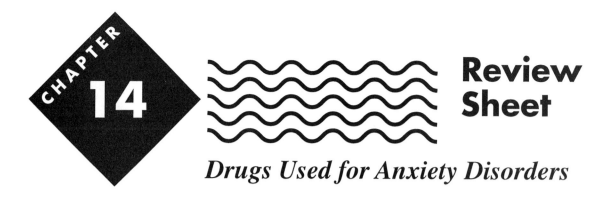

CHAPTER 14

Review Sheet

Drugs Used for Anxiety Disorders

The QUESTION column and the ANSWER column have been offset so that you can cover the answers while reading the questions, allowing you to assess your knowledge.

Question

1. Define *anxiety disorder*.
2. What is a *phobia*?

3. What is obsessive-compulsive disorder?

4. What is a panic disorder?

5. State another common name for *tranquilizers*.
6. Summarize nursing assessments and interventions that are used for the patient displaying anxiety.
7. State the action of benzodiazepines.
8. What is the ending spelling of all generic drug names of benzodiazepines except chlordiazepoxide?

9. Name three benzodiazepines that are relatively short acting and therefore most appropriate for an older adult or an individual with reduced hepatic function.
10. What premedication assessments should be performed prior to administering a benzodiazepine?

11. State the desired therapeutic outcome for any drug prescribed for an anxiety disorder.

Answer

1. Patients are said to suffer from an anxiety disorder when their responses to stressful situations are abnormal, irrational, and impair normal daily functioning.
2. Phobias are irrational fears of a specific object, activity, or situation. The patient recognizes the fear as exaggerated or unrealistic. The fear persists, however, and the patient seeks to avoid the situation.
3. An obsession is an unwanted thought, idea, image, or urge that a patient recognizes as time consuming and senseless but that repeatedly intrudes into the consciousness despite attempts to ignore, prevent, or counteract it. A compulsion is a repetitive, intentional, purposeful behavior performed to decrease the anxiety associated with an obsession.
4. See textbook, p. 192.
5. Tranquilizers are also called *anxiolytic agents* or *antianxiety* medications.
6. See textbook, pp. 193-194
7. Benzodiazepines stimulate an inhibitory neurotransmitter gamma amino benzoic acid (GABA).
8. All generic drug names of benzodiazepines end in "-pam."

9. Alprazolam, lorazepam, oxazepam are appropriate benzodiazepines for older adults or individuals with reduced hepatic function.
10. Before administering a benzodiazepine, assess for level of anxiety present; vital signs, especially blood pressure in sitting and supine positions; blood dyscrasias; hepatic disease; and whether the patient is in the first trimester of pregnancy or breast-feeding.

Copyright © 2001 by Mosby, Inc.   All rights reserved.

12. Why is the use of benzodiazepines avoided during the first trimester of pregnancy?

13. Describe side effects to expect with buspirone (BuSpar), hydroxyzine (Vistaril), and meprobamate (Equanil).

14. Based on the side effects of the drugs listed in question 11, what nursing diagnosis statements could be developed?

15. When you read a drug monograph that lists possible orthostatic hypotension as a side effect, what nursing actions would be appropriate, in addition to teaching the patient to rise slowly from a supine to sitting position?

16. What are additive effects associated with concurrent CNS system depressants?

17. What are symptoms of hepatotoxicity?

18. What are the side effects to expect with hydroxyzine?

19. What is the major advantage of buspirone, an azaspirone agent, over other antianxiety agents?

20. What is the action of fluvoxamine (Luvox), an SSRI agent?

21. When used as a preoperative medication, what are the desired actions of hydroxyzine (Vistaril, Atarax)?

11. The desired outcome of drug therapy for anxiety disorders is a decreased level of anxiety so that the individual can function normally in life's daily activities.

12. Use of benzodiazepines in the first trimester of pregnancy is associated with increased incidence of birth defects.

13. Side effects to expect include sedation and lethargy with buspirone; blurred vision, constipation, dryness of mucous membranes, and sedation with hydroxyzine; and sedation, slurred speech, and dizziness with meprobamate.

14. A possible nursing diagnosis is: Injury, high risk for, related to antianxiety drug therapy (meprobamate, buspirone, hydroxyzine) manifested by lethargy, sedation, blurred vision, dizziness.

15. Monitor blood pressure in supine and standing positions every shift and provide for patient safety.

16. Combining more than one drug that depresses the CNS will cause exaggeration of the depressant effects and could reach potentially fatal levels.

17. Symptoms of hepatotoxicity include anorexia, nausea, vomiting, hepatomegaly, splenomegaly, and abnormal liver function tests (elevated bilirubin, AST, ALT, GGT, alkaline phosphatase, and prothrombin time).

18. Side effects to expect with hydroxyzine include blurred vision, constipation, dry mucosa (thirst), and sedation.

19. There is lower incidence of sedation with buspirone.

20. Luvox inhibits serotonin reuptake at the nerve endings, prolonging the serotonin activity. It is used to assist persons with obsessive-compulsive disorder to gain better control over obsessive actions.

21. Used preoperatively, hydroxyzine causes sedation, acts as an antiemetic and reduces the narcotic dose needed for analgesia.

Copyright © 2001 by Mosby, Inc. All rights reserved.

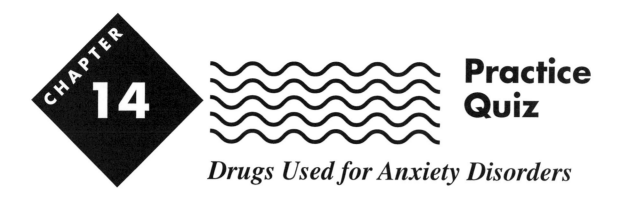

CHAPTER 14

Practice Quiz

Drugs Used for Anxiety Disorders

DEFINITIONS

Define the following terms:

1. Tranquilizer—

2. Compulsion—

3. Phobias—

4. Panic disorder—

5. Obsession—

6. Anxiety—

NURSING PROCESS

7. Summarize the nursing assessments used to collect data relating to:
   a. mood/affect

   b. clarity of thought

   c. psychomotor functions

   d. obsessions or compulsions

   e. sleep pattern

   f. dietary history

8. What is the nursing intervention with the highest priority for an individual suffering from a severe anxiety attack?

DRUG ACTIONS/SIDE EFFECTS

State the action and side effects of the following drug classes or drugs used in the treatment of anxiety disorders.

	Actions	*Side Effects*
9. Benzodiazepines		
10. Azaspirones		
11. Hydroxyzine		
12. Meprobamate		

13. What premedication assessments should be performed prior to administering a benzodiazepine?

ESSAY

Read the following situation and answer the questions.

Situation: J.H. enters the unit with symptoms of generalized anxiety disorder. During the admission interview the following information is obtained.

J.H. is so fearful of losing her job that she discusses the possibility several times a day. This has been an increasing concern over the past eight months. Her work performance was previously regarded as above average; however, over the past two months she has had increasing difficulty concentrating and completing her responsibilities. Finally, last week her employer suggested she take a brief vacation to "get it together." Since then her symptoms have escalated significantly.

   She is having difficulty falling asleep and frequently awakens with palpitations and clammy hands.

Copyright © 2001 by Mosby, Inc.   All rights reserved.

When asked to describe her feelings she says, "I'm out of control, I'm going to lose my job. What am I ever going to do?"

1. What additional nursing assessments must be made? Research a typical data intake assessment sheet used with anxiety disorder.
2. J.H.'s admission orders include giving alprazolam 0.25 mg, tid. What time schedule would be used to administer these doses?
3. Describe premedication assessment data needed and what additional assessments should be made after initiation of drug therapy using benzodiazepines.
4. How soon after initiation of drug therapy is it reasonable to expect a therapeutic response from antianxiety medication?
5. Describe the behavior monitoring system and intervention flow records used to detect the side effects of anxiolytic drugs in the clinical setting where you are assigned.
6. What assessments and nursing interventions (including health teaching) need to be performed to deal with the possible physical dependence or tolerance known to occur with benzodiazepine therapy?

END-OF-CHAPTER MATH REVIEW

1. Ordered: Hydroxyzine (Vistaril) 20 mg, IM, stat.
   On hand: Hydroxyzine (Vistaril) 25 mg/ml.
   Give: _____ ml.
2. Ordered: Meprobamate (Miltown) 1600 mg, po daily in four divided doses.
   How many mg/dose will be administered?
3. Ordered: Lorazepam (Ativan) 3 mg, IM, stat
   On hand: Lorazepam (Ativan) 4 mg/ml.
   Give: _____ ml.

Copyright © 2001 by Mosby, Inc. All rights reserved.

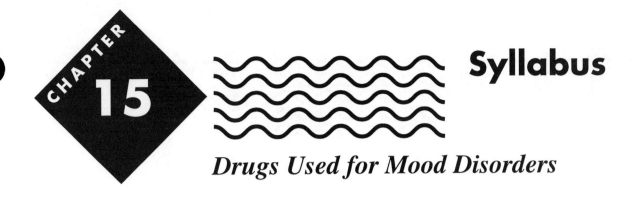

CHAPTER 15

Syllabus

Drugs Used for Mood Disorders

CHAPTER OBJECTIVES

1. Describe the essential components of a baseline assessment of a patient with depression or bipolar disorder.
2. Discuss the mood swings associated with bipolar disorder.
3. Compare drug therapy used during the treatment of the manic phase and depressive phase of bipolar disorder.
4. Cite monitoring parameters used for persons taking monoamine oxidase inhibitors (MAOIs), selective serotonin reuptake inhibitors (SSRIs), or tricyclic antidepressants.
5. Prepare a teaching plan for an individual receiving tricyclic antidepressants.
6. Differentiate between the physiologic and psychologic therapeutic responses seen with antidepressant therapy.
7. Identify premedication assessments necessary before administration of MAOIs, SSRIs, tricyclic antidepressants, and antimanic agents.
8. Compare the mechanism of action of SSRIs to that of other antidepressant agents.
9. Cite the advantages of SSRIs over other antidepressant agents.
10. Examine the monographs for SSRIs to identify significant drug interactions.

KEY WORDS

mood	mania
mood disorder	euphoria
depression	labile mood
neurotransmitter	grandiose
cognitive symptoms	delusion
psychomotor symptoms	suicide
bipolar disorder	antidepressant

ASSIGNMENTS

Read textbook, pp. 201-217.
Study Key Words associated with chapter content.
Study Review Sheet for Chapter 15.
Complete End-of-Chapter Math Review and Critical
    Thinking Questions.
Complete Collaborative Activity as assigned by instructor.
Complete Chapter 15 Practice Quiz.
Complete Chapter 15 Exam.

COLLABORATIVE ACTIVITIES

Complete the following research questions. Be prepared to share your findings during in-class discussion and group work that may be assigned by the instructor.

Research the type of monitoring that is performed to detect extrapyramidal symptoms (EPS) in the clinical site(s) where you are assigned.

1. What records and reports are used?
2. How often are the assessments performed and recorded?
3. When extrapyramidal symptoms are initially detected, what are the appropriate nursing actions?

Copyright © 2001 by Mosby, Inc. All rights reserved.

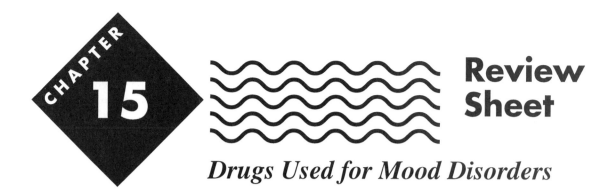

Review Sheet

Drugs Used for Mood Disorders

The QUESTION column and the ANSWER column have been offset so that you can cover the answers while reading the questions, allowing you to assess your knowledge.

Question	Answer
Question	**Answer**

Question

1. Define *mood disorders*.
2. Which neurotransmitters are affected by depression?

3. Define *bipolar disorder*.

4. Define *flight of ideas*.

5. Cite the incidence of attempted suicide in individuals with mood disorders.
6. Give two examples of cognitive symptoms and psychomotor symptoms.

7. Define *labile moods*.

8. Define *grandiose thinking*.

9. Describe basic components of assessment for an individual with a mood disorder.
10. In general, what is the decision making capacity of an individual with a mood disorder?

11. List the drug classifications used in the treatment of depression.

Answer

1. Mood disorders are also known as *affective disorders*. The person's ability to function is impaired for a prolonged period of time going beyond brief periods of emotional upset from negative life experiences. Mood disorders are characterized by abnormal feelings of euphoria and/or depression.
2. Norepinephrine, serotonin, and dopamine are the neurotransmitters affected by depression.
3. Bipolar disorder is characterized by distinct episodes of mania (euphoria) and depression separated by intervals without mood disturbances.
4. Quick thoughts that rapidly change from one topic to another is called flight of ideas.
5. The frequency of suicide attempts in individuals with mood disorders is 15%, 30 times higher than general population.
6. Cognitive symptoms involve the ability to concentrate, altered clarity of thought (e.g., confusion, poor short-term memory). Psychomotor symptoms include slowed or retarded movements, pacing, and outbursts of shouting.
7. Labile moods are rapid shifts in mood. A person may be happy, then rapidly switch to anger and irritability.
8. Grandiose thinking is overestimation of one's self and one's abilities or importance.
9. Basic components of assessment for mood disorders include history of mood disorders, basic mental status, interpersonal relationships, mood/affect, clarity of thought, thoughts of death, psychomotor function, sleep pattern, and dietary history.
10. The decision making capacity of an individual with a mood disorder is highly variable. The nurse must evaluate the individual's abilities and need to be protected from self-harm.

 Copyright © 2001 by Mosby, Inc.   All rights reserved.

12. What are the basic actions of medicines used to treat depression?

13. Why is it necessary to closely monitor patients taking antidepressants?

14. What is the anticipated therapeutic outcome for antidepressant therapy?

15. Discuss premedication assessments needed for an individual who is to receive 1) MAOIs, 2) SSRIs, 3) tricyclic antidepressants, or 4) miscellaneous agents, including bupropion, maprotiline, nefazodone, trazodone, and venlafaxine.

16. State appropriate nursing diagnoses as indicators of antidepressant therapy.

17. Name the drug used to treat manic episodes. List the important premedication assessments as well as assessments needed for long-term therapy.

18. List the normal serum level for lithium.

19. Describe teaching that should be completed about sodium intake while receiving lithium therapy.

20. Why is behavioral monitoring during antidepressant therapy done?

11. Drugs used in the treatment of depression include monoamine oxidase inhibitors (MAOIs), tricyclic antidepressants, selective serotonin reuptake inhibitors (SSRIs), and miscellaneous group of monocyclic and tetracyclic agents.

12. All antidepressants block the uptake and destruction of the neurotransmitters serotonin, norepinephrine, and/or dopamine.

13. Patients taking antidepressants may be suicidal. When drug therapy is initiated, it may take 1-4 weeks before a therapeutic response is evident. An early improvement in mood or other symptoms should not be used as an indicator that the depression is no longer present. Individuals may require 4-6 weeks to reach a full therapeutic level of the medicine.

14. The anticipated therapeutic outcome for individuals taking antidepressants is improvement of mood with a concurrent reduction in the feelings of depression.

15. MAOIs, textbook p. 207; SSRIs, textbook p. 209; tricyclic Antidepressants, p. 210; misc. agents textbook, p. 211.

16. Risk for violence: self-inflicted—hopelessness—dysfunctional grieving—ineffective individual coping—social isolation

17. Lithium carbonate (Eskalith, Lithane) is used to treat manic episodes. Before beginning lithium therapy, stress importance of the need for adequate hydration and sodium intake. Teach the patient the signs of lithium toxicity (e.g., nausea, vomiting, abdominal pain, diarrhea, lethargy, speech difficulty, mild dizziness, muscle twitching, and tremors).

18. Normal serum lithium range is 0.4 to 1.5 mEq/L.

19. During lithium therapy, normal daily intake of sodium is essential, as is adequate hydration. Stress using salt in cooking and at the table. The person should also drink 10-12 8 oz. glasses of water daily.

20. Behavioral monitoring during antidepressant therapy is done to detect development of extrapyramidal symptoms and to monitor for degree of therapeutic response to therapy.

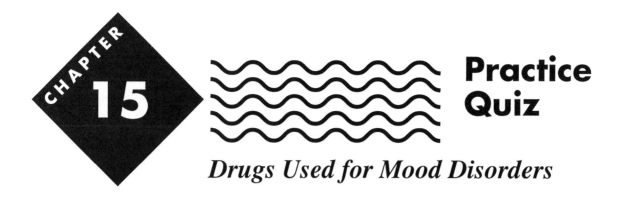

CHAPTER 15

Practice Quiz

Drugs Used for Mood Disorders

COMPLETION

Complete the following statements.

F.T. has been diagnosed with bipolar disorder. This disorder is characterized by mood swings between

1. _____, and
2. _____ (abnormal degree of sadness)

Drug classes known as antidepressants include:

3. _____
4. _____
5. _____
6. _____

Premedication assessments for MAOIs should include:

7. _____
8. _____
9. _____
10. _____

Behavioral monitoring is used to detect:

11. _____
12. _____
13. What is the generally recognized mechanism of action of antidepressant medications?

14. Persons taking MAOIs must omit foods containing:

15. Which classification of antidepressants is most widely used today in the treatment of depression?

16. A major bothersome side effect of tricyclic antidepressant therapy is:

Two additional common side effects of tricyclic antidepressants are:

17. _____, and
18. _____

Premedication assessments prior to initiation of lithium therapy should include:

19. _____
20. _____
21. _____
22. _____
23. The normal therapeutic range for serum lithium is:

ESSAY

1. During her clinic visit, R.S. complains to the nurse that since she started taking amitriptyline (Elavil) for depression, she has had a "terrible dry mouth" and she feels "sleepy all the time." What additional information would you elicit? What interventions to alleviate these symptoms could be suggested?

2. The next patient at the clinic is taking fluoxetine (Prozac) He is 5'6" tall, weighs 120 lbs. and has been receiving the medication for 6 weeks. He reports that he feels like a "cloud has been lifted from my mind." What additional data would be appropriate to collect during this visit?

3. When a patient is starting therapy with an MAOI, what health teaching is important?

4. The drug monograph for MAOI therapy states that one major potential complication of this therapy is hypertensive crisis. Discuss hypertensive crisis, how to recognize it, and the interventions that should be implemented if it occurs.

5. Discuss the behavioral monitoring sheets used in the clinical setting where you are practicing to assess for the development of extrapyramidal symptoms. How often are the assessments made, how are they recorded, and when is the physician notified of changes in the patient's behavior?

Copyright © 2001 by Mosby, Inc.   All rights reserved.

Situation (for questions 6–8): M.H., age 34, is being treated for bipolar disorder with lithium 300 mg, po, 4 times daily. She is being seen today in the clinic. During the intake interview she tells the nurse that her medicine "never works." Further exploration reveals that she has not taken the medication for the past 4 days.

6. When reviewing M.H.'s history, the nurse reads that her lithium level taken the month before was 2.0 mEq/L. As the nurse in this situation, how would you proceed?

7. What symptoms might you expect with this lithium level?

8. The history also notes that the importance of adequate intake of water and sodium was discussed with M.H. How does the sodium level within the body influence the metabolism of lithium?

END-OF-CHAPTER MATH REVIEW

1. Ordered: Lithium carbonate 300 mg, po, twice daily
   On hand: Lithium carbonate 150 mg tablets
   Give: _____ tablets

2. Ordered: Maprotiline 100 mg, po, this A.M.
   On hand: None found in medication container; consult drug monograph for dosage availability. What strength tablets would most likely be dispensed and how would you administer the dose?

Copyright © 2001 by Mosby, Inc. All rights reserved.

CHAPTER 16

Drugs Used for Psychoses

Syllabus

CHAPTER CONTENTS

CHAPTER OBJECTIVES

1. Identify signs and symptoms of psychosis.
2. Describe major indications for the use of antipsychotic agents.
3. Identify common adverse effects observed with antipsychotic medications.
4. Develop a teaching plan for a patient taking haloperidol and for a person receiving clozapine.

KEY WORDS

psychosis
delusions
hallucinations
disorganized thinking
loosening of associations
disorganized behavior
changes in affect
target symptoms
typical and atypical
    antipsychotic agents
equipotent doses
extrapyramidal symptoms
dystonia

pseudoparkinsonian
    symptoms
akathisia
tardive dyskinesia
abnormal involuntary
    movement scale
dyskinesia identification
    systems: condensed
    user scale
neuroleptic malignant
    syndrome
depot antipsychotic
    medicine

ASSIGNMENTS

Read textbook, pp. 217-225.
Study Key Words associated with chapter content.
Study Review Sheet for Chapter 16.
Complete End-of-Chapter Math Review and Critical Thinking Questions.
Complete Collaborative Activity, as assigned by instructor.
Complete Chapter 16 Practice Quiz.
Complete Chapter 16 Exam.

COLLABORATIVE ACTIVITIES

Complete the following activity and questions. Be prepared to share your findings during in-class discussion and group work that may be assigned by the instructor.

Perform an assessment of a patient receiving an antipsychotic medication, such as clozapine.
1. What laboratory studies were completed on admission or prior to initiating therapy?
2. Compare the laboratory studies performed in question 1 with the most recent laboratory values. Are there significant changes, and if so, what nursing actions would be appropriate?

    Are the recommended laboratory studies listed in the drug monograph, textbook p. 224, being performed? If not, what nursing actions would be appropriate?

Copyright © 2001 by Mosby, Inc.   All rights reserved.

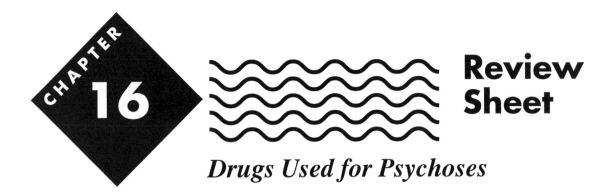

CHAPTER 16

Review Sheet

Drugs Used for Psychoses

The QUESTION column and the ANSWER column have been offset so that you can cover the answer while reading the questions, allowing you to assess your knowledge.

Question	Answer
1. Define *psychosis*.	
2. Differentiate between delusions, hallucinations, and disorganized thinking.	1. Psychosis does not have a single definition, but is a clinical descriptor that means that a person is out of touch with reality.
3. What is change in affect?	2. Delusions are false, irrational beliefs unchanged in the presence of data to the contrary. Hallucinations are false sensory perceptions experienced by an individual without external stimulus. Disorganized thinking is recognized when an individual switches rapidly from one idea or thought to another unrelated topic.
4. What is meant by *target symptoms*?	3. Change in affect is characterized by diminished emotional expression, reduced spontaneous movement, and poor eye contact. The individual withdraws from effective functioning in interpersonal relations, work, education, and self-care.
5. What are typical and atypical antipsychotic agents?	4. Target symptoms are those symptoms to be assessed to evaluate therapeutic response to drug therapy and nonpharmacologic interventions.
6. What is the general mechanism of action of antipsychotic agents?	5. Typical agents are listed in Table 16-1, p. 220. Atypical antipsychotic agents include clozapine, olanzapine, quetiapine, and risperidone. These classifications are based on the drugs' mechanisms of action. See textbook, pp. 219 for an explanation of the actions of antipsychotic agents on dopamine receptors.
7. Cite the desired therapeutic outcome(s) from antipsychotic therapy.	6. Antipsychotics antagonize the neurotransmitter dopamine in the CNS.
8. Define extrapyramidal symptoms, including dystonia, pseudoparkinsonian symptoms, akathisia, and tardive dyskinesia.	7. Calmed the individual, reduced psychomotor agitation and insomnia, reduced thought disorders so the individual is able to function with minimal exacerbation of psychotic symptoms.

Copyright © 2001 by Mosby, Inc. All rights reserved.

9. What causes pseudoparkinsonian symptoms?

10. What are the DISCUS or AIMS scales?

11. Describe common adverse effects associated with antipsychotic therapy.

12. What is neuroleptic malignant syndrome? What are the symptoms, and how is it treated?

13. Summarize nursing implementations and patient education used for patients being treated for psychoses.

14. Memorize the generic and brand names of these commonly prescribed antipsychotic agents: Thorazine, Trilafon, Mellaril, Clozaril, Haldol and Risperidal.

8. Dystonia is spasmodic movements of muscle groups (e.g., tongue protrusion, rolling back of the eyes). Pseudoparkinsonian symptoms are tremors, muscular rigidity, mask-like expression, shuffling gait, and loss or weakness of motor function. Akathisia is a feeling of anxiety, restlessness, pacing, rocking, and inability to sit still. Tardive dyskinesia is progressive symptoms of involuntary, hyperkinetic, abnormal movements.

9. Pseudoparkinsonian symptoms are caused by a relative deficiency of dopamine and an excess of acetylcholine, caused by antipsychotic agents.

10. Both the DISCUS and AIMS scales are involuntary movement scales for rating dyskinetic movements. (See Appendix G for the DISCUS scale.)

11. Adverse effects of antipsychotic therapy include sedation, drowsiness, appetite stimulation, postural hypotension, reflex tachycardia, lowering of seizure threshold, and development of symptoms of tardive dyskinesia.

12. See textbook. Symptoms of neuroleptic malignant syndrome include fever, extrapyramidal symptoms, and lead-pipe rigidity, probably due to excessive dopamine depletion. It is treated with bromocriptine or amantadine as dopamine agonists and dantrolene, a muscle relaxant. Fever is treated with cooling blankets, adequate hydration, and antipyretics.

13. See textbook, pp. 223-224.

14. The generic and brand names of commonly prescribed antipsychotic agents are: chlorpromazine, Thorazine; perphenazine, Trilafon; thioridazine, Mellaril; clozapine, Clozaril; and haloperidol, Haldol.

Copyright © 2001 by Mosby, Inc.   All rights reserved.

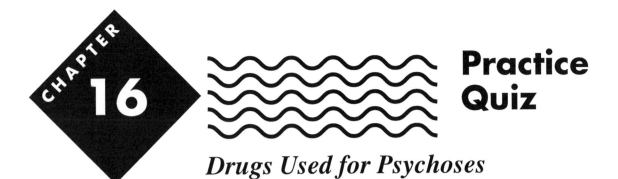

CHAPTER 16

Practice Quiz

Drugs Used for Psychoses

MATCHING

Select the definition that best describes the term(s) listed.

_____ 1. hallucin-
ations

_____ 2. delusions

_____ 3. akathisia

_____ 4. tardive
dyskinesia

_____ 5. dystonia

a. Syndrome demon-
strated by anxiety,
restlessness, pacing,
and rocking

b. Alternating feelings of
danger and elation

c. Involuntary hyperki-
netic abnormal
movements

d. False sensory percep-
tions being experi-
enced without external
stimulus

e. Prolonged spasmodic
movements of muscle
groups

ab. A false, irrational
belief that a patient
embraces despite
evidence to the
contrary

ESSAYS

J.S. is taking a high-potency antipsychotic medication.

6. What are high-potency antipsychotics and what drugs
are included in this category?

7. What are extrapyramidal side effects? How often
should the patient be monitored for these symptoms?
When found, what nursing actions are appropriate?

8. It is decided that J.S. should receive clozapine. What
are the side effects to expect and those to report with
this medication?

9. Discuss monitoring for agranulocytosis.

10. Why is an anticholinergic agent frequently given in
addition to haloperidol? What is its action?

11. State the usual anticipated side effects seen with
antipsychotic therapy.

12. Explain the behavioral monitoring system used in
your clinical site to detect extrapyramidal symptoms.

List the generic or brand names of the following
antipsychotic agents:

13. chlorpromazine

14. Trilafon

15. Mellaril

16. Clozapine

17. Haldol

END-OF-CHAPTER MATH REVIEW

1. The doctor orders chlorpromazine (Thorazine) 125
mg.
On hand is chlorpromazine 100 mg per 5 ml.
Give _____ ml.

2. The physician orders benztropine mesylate
(Cogentin) 1 mg, po, at bedtime daily. Available is
benztropine mesylate 0.5 mg tablets.
Give _____ tablets.

3. The physician orders trifluoperazine (Stelazine) 12
mg IM. On hand is trifluoperazine 10 mg/ml and 20
mg/ml. Which concentration would you use and what
volume should be injected?

Copyright © 2001 by Mosby, Inc. All rights reserved.

CHAPTER 17

Syllabus

Drugs Used for Seizure Disorders

CHAPTER CONTENT

CHAPTER OBJECTIVES

1. Prepare a chart to be used as a study guide that includes the following information:
   Name of seizure type
   Description of seizure
   Medications used to treat each type of seizure
   Nursing interventions and monitoring parameters for seizures
2. Describe the effects of the hydantoins on patients with diabetes and on persons receiving oral contraceptives, theophylline, folic acid, or antacids.
3. Cite precautions needed when administering phenytoin or diazepam intravenously.
4. Explain the rationale for proper dental care for persons receiving hydantoin therapy.
5. Develop a teaching plan for persons diagnosed with a seizure disorder.
6. Cite the desired therapeutic outcomes for drug therapy for seizure disorders.
7. Identify the mechanisms of action thought to control seizure activity when anticonvulsants are administered.
8. Discuss the basic classification system used to describe types of epilepsy.

KEY WORDS

seizures
epilepsy
partial seizures
anticonvulsants
tonic phase
clonic phase
postictal state
status epilepticus

atonic seizure
myoclonic seizures
absence (petit mal) epilepsy
seizure threshold
GABA
gingival hyperplasia
nystagmus

ASSIGNMENTS

Read textbook, pp. 226-239.
Study Key Words associated with chapter content.
Study Review Sheet for Chapter 17.
Complete End-of-Chapter Math Review and Critical Thinking Questions.
Complete Collaborative Activity as assigned by instructor.
Complete Chapter 17 Practice Quiz.
Complete Chapter 17 Exam.

COLLABORATIVE ACTIVITIES

Respond to the following case study. Be prepared to share your response during in-class discussion and group work that may be assigned by the instructor.

A.C. is receiving ethotoin (Peganone) 500 mg, po, qid. He is an insulin-dependent diabetic. What patient education should be performed when initiating this treatment and as the drug therapy progresses?

Copyright © 2001 by Mosby, Inc.   All rights reserved.

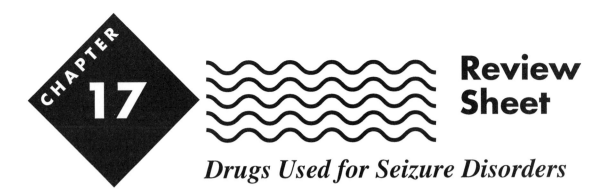
The QUESTION column and the ANSWER column have been offset so that you can cover the answer while reading the question, allowing you to assess your knowledge.

Question	**Answer**
1. Define *seizures*.	
2. List the four general types of epilepsy.	1. Seizures are brief periods of abnormal electrical activity in the brain that may or may not produce violent, involuntary muscle activity.
3. Differentiate among tonic phase, clonic phase, and postictal state.	2. The four general types of epilepsy are partial, generalized, unilateral, and unclassified (Figure 17-1, p. 228).
4. *Drop attack* is the layman's term for what kind of seizure?	3. Tonic phase is when patient has intense muscle contractions, loss of consciousness, and rigidity of the body. The clonic phase is characterized by alternating jerking and relaxation of the muscles of the extremities. The patient may defecate or urinate during this phase. The postictal period is the period immediately following a seizure, during which the patient rests. The patient has no recollection of the attack after awakening.
5. Differentiate between absence (petit mal) epilepsy and partial seizures.	4. Atonic seizures are characterized by a sudden loss of muscle tone, causing the head or limb to suddenly "drop." There is also loss of consciousness.
6. What assessments should the nurse make during seizure activity?	5. Petit mal seizures occur primarily in children. These seizures are characterized by a 5-20 second period of altered consciousness accompanied by a few rhythmic movements with no frank convulsive movements and no memory of events during the seizure. Partial seizures are localized convulsions of voluntary muscles. The person does not lose consciousness unless the partial seizure progresses into generalized seizure.
7. Name two barbiturates that are effective for anticonvulsant therapy.	6. During seizure activity, the nurse should note a description of the seizure, including onset, duration, body parts involved, any progression of symptoms, state of consciousness, respiratory pattern, salivation, pupil size and eye movement, and incontinence.
8. Name the three benzodiazepines used for anticonvulsant therapy.	7. Barbiturates that are effective for anticonvulsive therapy include phenobarbital and mephobarbital.

Copyright © 2001 by Mosby, Inc.   All rights reserved.

9. Review the side effects of benzodiazepines.

10. What premedication assessments should be done before beginning hydantoin therapy?
11. What assessments need to be performed when a diabetic patient is taking hydantoins?

12. What specific drug classified as a hydantoin is NEVER mixed in the same syringe with other medications?
13. List the signs and symptoms of phenytoin toxicity.

14. What is a brand name of phenytoin?

15. What over-the-counter drug decreases the therapeutic effects of hydantoins?
16. Phenytoin reduces the serum levels of disopyramide and quinidine; therefore, the nurse should monitor for what?
17. Phenytoin may interfere with oral contraception. What measures need to be implemented to prevent pregnancy?
18. Theophylline derivative drugs interact with phenytoin, which often requires increases in the theophylline dosages. What symptoms would indicate such an interaction is occurring?
19. What is the fourth class of drugs used to treat seizures?

20. Carbamazepine (Tegretol) may be used in combination with other anticonvulsant agents. What laboratory studies are recommended with its use?
21. What patient education should be given to patients taking phenytoin and oral contraceptives?

22. What over-the-counter drugs can decrease the therapeutic effectiveness of phenytoin?

23. Analyze the drug monograph for hydantoins and describe the patient education needed.
24. What is the action of lamotrigine (Lamictal)?
25. Why is it necessary to check on whether a patient is already taking valproic acid before initiating therapy with lamotrigine?

8. Benzodiazepines used for anticonvulsant therapy include diazepam (Valium), clonazepam (Klonopin), and clorazepate (Tranxene). See also Table 17-1.
9. Side effects of benzodiazepines include drowsiness, lethargy, dizziness, fatigue, ataxia, and blurred vision.
10. Before beginning hydantoin therapy, review routine blood studies to detect blood dyscrasias and hepatotoxicity. For diabetics, obtain a baseline serum glucose level. Because hydantoins can cause mental confusion, baseline mental status data should be assessed before starting these agents.
11. Persons who are diabetics need regular checks for hyperglycemia while taking hydantoins.
12. Phenytoin (Dilantin) is never mixed in the same syringe with other medications.
13. Signs and symptoms of phenytoin toxicity include nystagmus, sedation, and lethargy.
14. Dilantin is the brand name of phenytoin.

15. Antacids decrease the therapeutic effects of hydantoins.

16. The nurse should monitor for cardiac arrhythmias during phenytoin therapy.

17. While receiving phenytoin, the patient should use an alternate contraceptive (e.g., diaphragm, foam, condoms).

18. Phenytoin decreases serum theophylline levels. Theophylline derivatives are bronchodilators; therefore, respiratory symptoms such as wheezing may occur if the drug's blood level is reduced.
19. The fourth class of drugs used to treat seizures is succinimides.

20. During carbamazepine therapy, complete blood count (CBC), liver function, urinalysis, BUN, serum creatinine, and ophthalmic tests should be performed.
21. Patients taking phenytoin and oral contraceptives concurrently should know to use another form of birth control if vaginal spotting or bleeding develops, and to consult a physician for possible adjustments in oral contraceptive dosage.
22. Antacids can decrease the therapeutic effects of phenytoin.
23. See textbook pp. 233-234.
24. Lamotrigine blocks voltage-sensitive sodium channels in neuronal membranes.

25. Approximately 10% of patients receiving lamotrigine develop a skin rash and urticaria in the first 4 to 6 weeks of therapy. Combination therapy with valproic acid appears to be more likely to precipitate a serious rash. (See textbook, p. 236.)

Copyright © 2001 by Mosby, Inc. All rights reserved.

Practice Quiz

Drugs Used for Seizure Disorders

COMPLETION

Complete the following statements.

1. Name four classifications of drugs used to treat seizure disorders.

2. What is the mechanism of action of anticonvulsants?

3. Describe the tonic and clonic phases of seizure activity.

4. Diazepam, clonazepam, and clorazepate are anticonvulsants classified as _____.

5. Phenytoin can cause _____ in a diabetic patient.

6. Alternatives to oral contraceptives should be used when a patient takes _____,
   _____, or _____ as an anticonvulsant.

7. A decrease in therapeutic effectiveness of phenytoin can occur when an OTC _____ is taken concurrently.

8. Summarize patient education that should be completed when a patient receives anticonvulsant therapy.

9. Describe side effects to report when carbamazepine (Tegretol) is administered.

END-OF-CHAPTER MATH REVIEW

1. Dr. Frye wrote orders to start J.B. on Dilantin 100 mg, tid and hs. What is your interpretation of the order and how will you administer it?

2. Dr. Haycock wrote orders to start B.S., a 10-year-old patient, on Tegretol suspension 50 mg, qid. The suspension is 100 mg/5ml. How will you administer this dose?

3. Dr. Tindall wrote orders for J.S., a 12-year-old, newly diagnosed epileptic weighing 110 lbs, to be started on Depakene syrup 5 ml, tid. The normal starting dose is 15 mg/kg daily. Is Dr. Tindall's order reasonable, and if so, how would you administer it?

CRITICAL THINKING QUESTIONS

1. Both Valium and Dilantin have very specific administration precautions when these agents are administered intravenously. What are these precautions?

2. R.C. suddenly had a tonic-clonic seizure while attending a class at college. When his family was notified of this and his need for transportation home, his wife tells you he has not been taking his medications regularly. Describe how you would address this situation.

3. While you are working in the emergency room, the rescue squad notifies the ER desk that a patient in status epilepticus is being transported. What medicines and equipment should you have ready for the patient's arrival?

4. What health teaching should be done for an individual recently diagnosed with epilepsy?

Copyright © 2001 by Mosby, Inc.   All rights reserved.

Syllabus

Drugs Used for Pain Management

CHAPTER CONTENT

CHAPTER OBJECTIVES

1. Differentiate among opiate agonists, opiate partial agonists, and opiate antagonists.
2. Describe monitoring parameters necessary for patients receiving opiate agonists.
3. Cite the side effects to expect when opiate agonists are administered.
4. Compare the analgesic effectiveness of opiate partial agonists when administered before or after opiate agonists.
5. Explain when naloxone can be used effectively to treat respiratory depression.
6. State the three pharmacologic effects of salicylates.
7. Prepare a list of side effects to expect, side effects to report, and drug interactions that are associated with salicylates.
8. Explain why synthetic nonopiate analgesics are not used for inflammatory disorders.
9. Prepare a patient education plan for a person being discharged with a continuing prescription for an analgesic.
10. Examine Table 18-4 and identify the active ingredients in commonly prescribed analgesic combination products. List products containing aspirin and compare the analgesic properties of agents available in different strengths.

KEY WORDS

pain experience
pain perception
pain threshold
pain tolerance
nociceptive pain
somatic pain
visceral pain
neuropathic pain
idiopathic pain
analgesics
opiate agonists
opiate partial agonists
opiate antagonists
nonsteroidal anti-
    inflammatory agents
nociceptors
opiate receptors
addiction
drug tolerance
ceiling effect
salicylates

ASSIGNMENTS

Read textbook, pp. 240-263.
Study Key Words associated with chapter content.
Study Review Sheet for Chapter 18.
Complete End-of-Chapter Math Review and Critical
    Thinking Questions.
Complete Collaborative Activity as assigned by instructor.
Complete Chapter 18 Practice Quiz.
Complete Chapter 18 Exam.

COLLABORATIVE ACTIVITIES

Complete the following activities and questions to prepare for in-class discussion and group work that may be assigned by the instructor.

1. Use a PDR or similar drug information reference available in the classroom or library to answer the following questions related to analgesics.
   a. What are the active ingredients of Empirin with Codeine?
   b. How does Empirin with Codeine No. 3 differ from Empirin with Codeine No. 4?
   c. What are the active ingredients in Tylenol with Codeine Nos. 2, 3, and 4?
   d. Compare the ingredients of Phenaphen with Tylenol with Codeine Nos. 3 and 4.
   e. What active ingredient does Percodan-Demi have that Percodan does not have?

Copyright © 2001 by Mosby, Inc. All rights reserved.

f. State the difference between the ingredients of Darvon Compound 65 and Darvon N.

g. If a patient is allergic to aspirin, which analgesic preparations can be used safely?

2. Develop charting for analgesic recording on inventory control sheet and prn medication record. Do all charting associated with administration of:

a. MS Contin 30 mg, po, at 8:15 A.M. today to:
   T.G., Rm. 611
   012-12-1234
   Dr. Martin
   Dx: Prostatic cancer with metastasis

b. Give T.G. Percodan, 1 tablet, at 10:15 A.M. today.

MEDICATION ADMINISTRATION RECORD

NAME:	RM-BD:	Init	Signature	Title
ID NO.:	AGE:			
DIAGNOSIS:	SEX:			

| PHYSICIAN: | Ht: | Wt: |

SCHEDULED MEDICATIONS

DATE	MEDICATION-STRENGTH-FORM-ROUTE	0030-0729	0730-1529	1530-0029

** PRN MEDICATIONS**				

Copyright © 2001 by Mosby, Inc.   All rights reserved.

CHAPTER

18

~~~~~~~~

Review Sheet

Drugs Used for Pain Management

The QUESTION column and the ANSWER column have been offset so that you can cover the answer while reading the questions, allowing you to assess your knowledge.

Question

1. Define *pain perception*, *pain threshold*, and *pain tolerance*.
2. Compare nociceptive pain, somatic pain, visceral pain, neuropathic pain, and idiopathic pain.

3. What neurotransmitters are known to stimulate nociceptors?

4. What are the four types of opiate receptors?

5. What drug is usually prescribed for severe, chronic pain?

6. Summarize nursing process for pain management.

7. Describe components of the McGill-Melzack pain questionnaire.
8. Describe patient education needed for an individual requiring long-term pain management.
9. Define *analgesic*.

10. What are agonists, antagonists, and partial agonists?
11. Opiate agonists are subdivided into what four groups?

Answer

1. Pain perception is awareness of the pain sensation. Pain threshold is the point at which pain is felt. Pain tolerance is an individual's ability to withstand the pain experience.
2. Nociceptive pain is a result of stimulus to pain receptors (dull, aching); somatic pain originates in the skin, bone, or muscle; visceral pain originates in the organs of the thorax or abdomen; neuropathic pain results from injury to the peripheral or central nervous systems; and idiopathic pain is of unknown origin.
3. The neurotransmitters bradykinin, prostaglandins, leukotrienes, histamines, and serotonin sensitize nociceptors.
4. The four types of opiate receptors are mu, delta, kappa, and sigma receptors. See textbook, p. 241 for further detailed discussion.
5. Morphine sulfate is usually prescribed for severe, chronic pain. It may also be combined with other drugs such as antidepressants.
6. See textbook, pp. 242-246.

7. See Figure 8-1, textbook pp. 243.

8. See textbook, pp. 246.

9. Analgesics are drugs that relieve pain.
10. Agonists interact with receptors to stimulate response. Antagonists attach to a receptor but do not stimulate a response or block a response. Partial agonists are drugs that interact with a receptor to stimulate a response, but may inhibit other responses.

Copyright © 2001 by Mosby, Inc. All rights reserved.

12. Identify pain assessment data needed to establish a baseline for monitoring therapy before initiating treatment for pain.

13. What is the most effective route for administering an analgesic when immediate relief is needed?
14. Explain the benefits of patient-controlled analgesia (PCA).
15. For what type(s) of pain are opiate agonists used?

16. What premedication assessments should be performed before administering an opiate agonist?
17. Will naloxone reverse CNS depression caused by sedative/hypnotics or tranquilizers?

18. When is naloxone effective?

19. What three drugs are antidotes for opiate agonists and opiate partial agonists?
20. Do opiate partial agonists relieve pain effectively in persons who have recently taken opiate agonists?
21. Give an example of an opiate partial agonist.

22. What are *physical dependence* and *tolerance*?
23. What is the most common drug used as an analgesic for relief of mild to moderate pain?

24. What three pharmacologic effects are associated with the salicylates?
25. When is ASA (aspirin) indicated?

26. What is salicylism?

27. What is the antidote for salicylism?

28. What are premedication assessments to perform before administering NSAIDs?

29. What are nonsteroidal anti-inflammatory drugs (NSAIDs)?
30. How do NSAIDs act?

11. Opiate agonists are divided into four groups: morphine-like derivatives, meperidine-like derivatives, methadone-like derivatives, and other opiate agonists.
12. Refer to text p. 243 for the McGill-Melzack pain questionnaire (Figure 18-2) for pain rating scales.
13. The intravenous route gives the most immediate pain relief.
14. With PCA, the patient can initiate the administration of analgesics, allowing pain relief to be obtained rapidly. Most important is the sense of control a patient feels toward the pain and scheduling daily activities. The PCA system monitors the total dose(s) administered and limits can be set on the total amount that can be self-administered during a specified period.
15. Opiate agonists are used for moderate to severe pain.

16. Baseline vital signs, neurologic exam, prior analgesics administered, and degree of pain control; voiding and bowel pattern.
17. Naloxone will not reverse CNS depression caused by sedative/hypnotics or tranquilizers.
18. Naloxone reverses the CNS depressant effects of the opiate agonists.
19. Nalmefene, naloxone, and naltrexone are antidotes for opiate agonists and opiate partial agonists.
20. Opiate partial agonists usually do not alleviate pain in persons who have recently taken opiate agonists.
21. See Table 18-2, p. 251.
22. Physical dependence means symptoms are controlled as long as daily opiate agonist requirements are met (addiction). Tolerance occurs when increased doses are required to achieve the same degree of pain relief.
23. Aspirin is the most common drug used to relieve mild to moderate pain.
24. Three pharmacologic effects of salicylates are analgesic, antipyretic, and anti-inflammatory.
25. ASA is indicated for analgesic effect, fever reduction, and anti-inflammatory effects. Do not give aspirin to children who may be developing a viral infection. Salicylates have been associated with Reye's syndrome.
26. Salicylism is seen with high doses of salicylates. Symptoms include tinnitus, impaired hearing, sweating, dizziness, mental confusion, and nausea and vomiting.
27. There is no antidote for salicylism. Use gastric lavage, force IV fluids, and alkalization of urine with IV sodium bicarbonate; stop salicylates.
28. See textbook, p. 259.

29. NSAIDs are a relatively new class of analgesics that includes aspirin.

Copyright © 2001 by Mosby, Inc.   All rights reserved.

31. Do NSAIDs control fever?

32. What is the major adverse effect of NSAIDs?

33. Name five commonly used NSAIDs.

34. Name the synthetic nonopiate analgesic used frequently for mild to moderate pain.
35. Compare the action of the drug in question 34 with the action of aspirin.

36. What are early indications of acetaminophen toxicity?
37. What premedication assessments are required for each classification of drug used to treat pain?

38. What effect does aspirin have on phenytoin, valproic acid, and oral hypoglycemic agents?

30. NSAIDs are prostaglandin inhibitors that have analgesic, anti-inflammatory and, in some cases (e.g., ibuprofen), antipyretic activity.
31. The antipyretic activity of most NSAIDs is low enough that they are not used clinically for fever control. Ibuprofen, however, is a good antipyretic agent and approved as such.
32. The major adverse effect of NSAID therapy is gastrointestinal (GI) complaints, which can develop into ulcers and GI bleeding.
33. See Table 18-3, p. 257.

34. Acetaminophen (Tylenol, Datril, Tempra) is a synthetic nonopiate analgesic used frequently for mild to moderate pain.
35. Acetaminophen has no anti-inflammatory effect. However, it is a very good antipyretic and analgesic.
36. Early indications of acetaminophen toxicity include nausea, anorexia, vomiting, and jaundice accompanied by an elevation in liver function tests.
37. This information can be found in sections listed as premedication assessments throughout Chapter 18.
38. When taken with aspirin, phenytoin levels are increased, causing toxicity: nystagmus, lethargy, sedation. Dosage adjustment may be required. Valproic acid levels are increased when taken with aspirin; dose adjustment may be needed. With oral hypoglycemics, aspirin increases potential for hypoglycemia.

Copyright © 2001 by Mosby, Inc.   All rights reserved.

Practice Quiz

Drugs Used for Pain Management

Define the following terms.
1. Pain perception

2. Pain threshold

3. Analgesic

4. List data needed prior to administering an analgesic:

5. List premedication assessments needed for an individual receiving an opiate agonist:

6. Are opiate partial agonists effective for pain management in an individual who has recently received an opiate agonist?

7. What are the side effects to expect with the administration of opiate agonists?

8. When should the drug naloxone (Narcan) be available?

9. List common side effects associated with salicylates.

10. Is acetaminophen (Tylenol) recommended for its anti-inflammatory properties?

Ordered: 1000 ml 5% D/W to run IV over the next 12 hours using a 15 gtt/ml administration set.

11. The IV should be adjusted to _____ gtt/min or
12. _____ ml/ hr.
13. When can acetaminophen be harmful to a patient?

14. What is salicylate overdose called and what are its signs and symptoms?

15. What drugs are used as antidotes for opiate agonists and opiate partial agonists?

END-OF-CHAPTER MATH REVIEW

1. Ordered: aspirin 650 mg, qid.
   On hand: aspirin 325 mg tablets.
   Give _____ tablets.
2. The pediatrician orders a 75 mg dose of ibuprofen suspension for a child. On hand is 100 mg/5 ml. Give _____ ml.
3. Morphine 15 mg IV every 6 hours has been ordered. Concentrations of 3, 4, 5, 8, 10, and 15 mg/ml are available. Which concentration would you use and what volume should be injected?
4. Dr. Sandmann wrote orders to start K.P. on codeine 30 mg qid after her wisdom tooth extraction. What is your interpretation of the order and how will you administer it?

CRITICAL THINKING QUESTIONS

1. F.C., a terminal cancer patient, returns to the unit with a morphine PCA pump going. His daughter comes to you alarmed that her father may "overuse" the morphine and become addicted. How would you respond to her? Give the rationale for your answer.
2. What is the difference between an order for morphine sulfate immediate release (MSIR) and an order for MS Contin?
3. P.T., age 86, is taking enteric-coated aspirin for her arthritis. She reports to the nurse that she thinks she saw a whole tablet in her stools. What followup would you do? She has been on continuous aspirin therapy for two years. Explain assessments needed.
4. The head nurse sends the student nurse to evaluate M.S.'s postoperative pain. Upon entering the patient's room, the student observes M.S. conversing and joking with her friends. The student decides not to further investigate the question of postoperative pain. Evaluate the correctness of the student's decision and give your rationale.

Copyright © 2001 by Mosby, Inc.   All rights reserved.

Syllabus

Drugs Used to Treat Hyperlipidemias

CHAPTER CONTENT

Atherosclerosis (p. 264)
Treatment of Hyperlipidemias (p. 265)
Drug Therapy for Hyperlipidemias (p. 265)
    Drug Class: Bile Acid-Binding Resins (p. 266)
    Drug Class: Niacin (p. 267)
    Drug Class: HMG-CoA Reductase Inhibitors (p. 268)
    Drug Class: Fibric Acids (p. 269)

CHAPTER OBJECTIVES

1. Identify the four major types of lipoproteins.
2. Describe the primary treatment modalities for lipid disorders.
3. State specific oral administration instructions needed with antilipidemic agents.
4. Analyze Table 19-1 to identify the specific agents used to treat type II and type IV forms of hyperlipidemia.

KEY WORDS

atherosclerosis
hyperlipidemia
triglycerides
lipoproteins
chylomicrons

ASSIGNMENTS

Read textbook, pp. 264-269.
Study Key Words associated with chapter content.
Study Review Sheet for Chapter 19.
Complete End-of-Chapter Math Review and Critical Thinking Questions.
Complete Collaborative Activity as assigned by instructor.
Complete Chapter 19 Practice Quiz.
Complete Chapter 19 Exam.

Copyright © 2001 by Mosby, Inc.   All rights reserved.

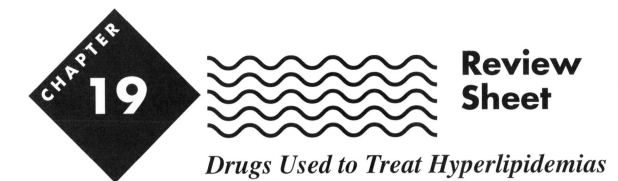

CHAPTER 19

Review Sheet

Drugs Used to Treat Hyperlipidemias

The QUESTION column and the ANSWER column have been offset so that you can cover the answer while reading the questions, allowing you to assess your knowledge.

Question

1. Define *atherosclerosis, hyperlipidemia, chylomicrons, triglycerides,* and *lipoproteins.*
2. What lifestyle changes should be used to treat hyperlipidemia prior to starting drug therapy?
3. Summarize nursing assessments needed for a patient with hyperlipidemia.

4. Why are supplemental vitamins required with bile acid-sequestering resins?

5. What are the signs and symptoms of a vitamin K deficiency?
6. Describe the proper preparation of cholestyramine for administration.

7. What drug interactions can occur with the use of bile-sequestering resins?

8. What is the primary desired therapeutic outcome from niacin?

9. What premedication assessments should be performed before administration of niacin?

Answer

1. See textbook, p. 264.

2. Lifestyle changes should be attempted for treatment of hyperlipidemia before starting drug therapy, including dietary changes (e.g., fat intake less than 30% of calories, decreased cholesterol and saturated fat intake, increased polyunsaturated and monounsaturated fats), weight reduction, and regular exercise.

3. Nursing assessments needed for patients with hyperlipidemia include risk factors (e.g., family history of increased cholesterol and lipids), smoking, dietary habits, glucose intolerance, elevated serum lipids, obesity, and sedentary lifestyle.

4. Bile-acid sequestering resins may deplete the body of its needed supply of fat-soluble vitamins (DEAK).

5. Bruising, bleeding gums, dark tarry stools, and "coffee ground" emesis are signs and symptoms of a vitamin K deficiency.

6. To prepare cholestyramine for administration, mix powdered resin with 2-6 oz water, soup, juice, or crushed pineapple; allow to stand until drug is absorbed and dispersed. Follow with an additional glass of water.

7. Bile-sequestering resins bind to a number of drugs such as digitoxin, warfarin, thyroxine, thiazide diuretics, NSAIDs, and beta blockers, and therefore reduce absorption of these drugs. Minimize this effect by administering 1 hour before or 4 hours after giving a resin. (See also textbook p. 267.)

8. The primary desired therapeutic outcome of niacin is decreased LDL and total cholesterol, decreased triglycerides, and increased HDL levels.

 Copyright © 2001 by Mosby, Inc. All rights reserved.

10. Name three statin drugs.

11. How long is the trial period used to evaluate the use of statins for hyperlipidemias?
12. What are common side effects to expect from antilipidemic therapy?
13. What anticipated alterations may occur in the blood glucose level with gemfibrozil?

9. Before administering niacin, assess serum triglyceride and cholesterol levels, liver function, baseline uric acid and blood glucose levels, and vital signs, and carefully document existing gastrointestinal symptoms.
10. The statin drugs include atorvastatin, fluvastatin, lovastatin, pravastatin, cervistatin, and simvastatin.
11. The trial period used to evaluate the use of statins for hyperlipidemias is a period of up to three months.
12. Nausea, diarrhea, flatulence, bloating, and abdominal distress are side effects to expect with antilipidemic therapy.
13. Gemfibrozil may cause moderate hyperglycemia.

Copyright © 2001 by Mosby, Inc. All rights reserved.

Practice Quiz

Drugs Used to Treat Hyperlipidemias

1. Name two -statin drugs used for hyperlipidemia.

2. What four primary therapeutic outcomes are expected from drug therapy for hyperlipidemia?

3. What effect does gemfibrozil have on blood glucose?

4. What premedication assessments should be completed prior to starting hyperlipidemia therapy?

5. What vitamins are affected by the administration of bile-sequestering drugs?

6. Knowing that digitalis and warfarin medications may be bound to bile-acid binding resins, what signs and symptoms should be assessed in the patient?

END-OF-CHAPTER MATH REVIEW

1. Ordered: Nicotinic acid (niacin) 1.5 g, po, in 3 divided doses daily.
   On hand: Nicotinic acid (niacin) 500 mg tablets
   Give: _____ tablets per dose
   A total of _____ mg daily

2. Ordered: Lovastatin (Mevacor) 80 mg, po, daily
   On hand: Lovastatin (Mevacor) 20 mg tablets
   Give: _____ tablets

CRITICAL THINKING QUESTIONS

1. Why is it essential to monitor a patient taking a bile-sequestering medication for a fat-soluble vitamin deficiency?

2. Why would bleeding problems be a potential side effect of bile-sequestering hypolipidemic drugs?

3. What effect do HMG-CoA reductase inhibitors have on LDL, HDL, VLDL cholesterol, and plasma triglycerides?

    When initiating therapy with a bile-acid binding resin, what assessments would be essential with regard to medications already prescribed?

Copyright © 2001 by Mosby, Inc.   All rights reserved.

Syllabus

Drugs Used to Treat Hypertension

CHAPTER CONTENT

CHAPTER OBJECTIVES

1. Summarize nursing assessments and interventions used during the treatment of hypertension.
2. State lifestyle modifications that should be implemented when a diagnosis of hypertension is made.
3. Identify the nine classes of drugs used to treat hypertension.
4. Review Figure 20-1 to identify options for, and progression of, treatment for hypertension.
5. Identify specific factors the hypertensive patient can use to assist in the management of the disease.
6. Develop objectives for patient education for patients with hypertension.
7. Summarize the mechanism of action of each drug class used to treat hypertension.

KEY WORDS

arterial blood pressure
systolic blood pressure
diastolic blood pressure
pulse pressure
mean arterial pressure
cardiac output
hypertension
primary hypertension
secondary hypertension

ASSIGNMENTS

Read textbook, pp. 271-291.
Study Key Words associated with chapter content.
Study Review Sheet for Chapter 20.
Complete End-of-Chapter Math Review and Critical Thinking Questions.
Complete Collaborative Activity, as assigned.
Complete Chapter 20 Practice Quiz.
Complete Chapter 20 Exam.

COLLABORATIVE ACTIVITY

Answer the following questions. Be prepared to share your responses during in-class discussion and group work that may be assigned by the instructor.

1. The nurse's aide asks you to explain why it is necessary to check a patient's blood pressure in the sitting, lying, and standing positions. What explanation is appropriate?
2. The next day, the nurse examines the blood pressures of a patient monitored q shift in sitting, lying, and standing positions yesterday. They are listed as:

BP	Sitting	Lying	Standing
7-3	140/90	140/90	140/90
3-11	156/96	160/94	164/92
11-7	156/84	142/80	158/86

What actions are appropriate based on this data?

Copyright © 2001 by Mosby, Inc. All rights reserved.

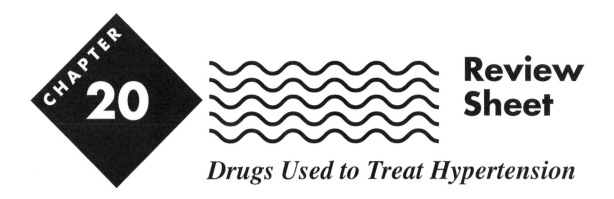

CHAPTER 20

Review Sheet

Drugs Used to Treat Hypertension

The QUESTION column and the ANSWER column have been offset so that you can cover the answer while reading the questions, allowing you to assess your knowledge.

Question

1. What are systolic and diastolic blood pressure?
2. How do you compute the mean arterial pressure or average pressure present throughout the heart cycle?

3. What are the primary determinants of systolic and diastolic blood pressure?
4. What is the definition of *hypertension*?

5. Differentiate between primary hypertension and secondary hypertension.

6. List the primary drug classifications used in the treatment of hypertension.

7. List the secondary drug classifications used in the treatment of hypertension.

8. What is the primary action of all antihypertensive drugs?

9. What is therapeutic outcome for antihypertensive therapy?
10. How does Joint National Commission (JNC) VI classify antihypertensive agents in current use?

Answer

1. Systolic blood pressure is pressure exerted as blood is pumped from the heart; diastolic blood pressure is the pressure present during the resting phase of the heartbeat.
2. See textbook, p. 271.

3. The primary determinant of systolic blood pressure is cardiac output, while the determinant for diastolic blood pressure is peripheral vascular resistance.
4. Hypertension is an elevation in either the systolic or diastolic blood pressure or both. See textbook, p. 272 for discussion of recommended screening in adults.
5. Primary hypertension is a controllable but not curable form of hypertension of unknown etiology. There are known risk factors that contribute to the development of primary hypertension. Secondary hypertension occurs following the development of another disorder in the body (e.g., renal disease, head trauma).
6. Hypertension is treated primarily with diuretics, beta-adrenergic blockers, angiotensin-converting enzyme (ACE) inhibitors, angiotensin II receptor antagonists, calcium ion antagonists, $alpha_1$ adrenergic blockers, central-acting $alpha_2$ agonists, peripheral-acting adrenergic antagonists, and direct vasodilators.
7. Secondary drug classifications used to treat hypertension include centrally acting $alpha_2$ agonists, peripherally acting adrenergic antagonists, and direct vasodilators.
8. The primary action of all antihypertensive drugs is to reduce BP and maintain it below 140/90 mm Hg.
9. The therapeutic outcome for antihypertensive therapy is lower blood pressure by reducing peripheral resistance.

Copyright © 2001 by Mosby, Inc.   All rights reserved.

11. What classification of drugs is used initially in the treatment of uncomplicated hypertension when lifestyle changes are not effective?
12. What is the treatment algorithm used for hypertension?

13. Describe the nursing process used for treatment of hypertension.
14. What are the nutritional goals for the treatment of hypertension?
15. Summarize the premedication assessments used prior to administration of antihypertensive drugs. (Examine differences between the various types of agents usually prescribed.)

16. What are the three classes of diuretic agents used to treat hypertension?
17. What laboratory test is used as a guide for when a patient needs to switch from a thiazide-type to a loop diuretic?
18. What are the major side effects to expect and report with beta-adrenergic blocking agents?

19. What types of patients should avoid the use of beta-blocking agents?

20. What precautions should be instituted when beta-blocker therapy is to be discontinued?

21. What effect does angiotensin II have on blood vessels?

22. What effect does an increase in aldosterone secretion have on blood pressure?
23. Summarize the side effects to expect and to report with the use of ACE inhibitors.

24. What is the action of angiotensin II receptor antagonists?

25. What are side effects to expect with alpha$_1$ adrenergic blockers?

26. Why should centrally acting alpha$_2$ agonists (e.g., clonidine, guanabenz, guanfacine, methyldopa) be discontinued gradually?

10. See textbook, pp. 273.

11. Drugs classified as diuretics and beta-adrenergic blocking agents are used initially in the treatment of uncomplicated hypertension.
12. See Figure 20-01, p. 274.

13. See textbook, pp. 276-277.

14. The nutritional goals for the treatment of hypertension include reduced sodium for most patients and a low-fat, low-calorie diet. Avoid lipids, saturated fats, caffeine, and alcohol, and eat foods high in potassium and calcium.
15. See multiple sections labeled premedication assessments throughout Chapter 20; e.g., pp. 278-279.
16. The three classes of diuretic agents used to treat hypertension are thiazide and thiazide-like agents, loop diuretics, and potassium-sparing diuretics.
17. The creatinine clearance test is used when a patient needs to switch from a thiazide-like to a loop diuretic.
18. The major side effects to expect and report with beta-adrenergic agents include bradycardia, peripheral vasoconstriction, bronchospasm, wheezing, hypoglycemia in diabetic patients, and heart failure.
19. Beta-blocking agents are not as effective in African-American patients and should be avoided in patients with asthma, type 1 diabetes mellitus, heart failure with an etiology of systolic dysfunction, and in patients with peripheral vascular disease.
20. After long-term treatment with beta blockers, discontinue gradually over 1 to 2 weeks and monitor for anginal symptoms.
21. Angiotensin II produces vasoconstriction, which results in an increase in blood pressure.
22. Aldosterone results in sodium retention, which causes increased cardiac output, thereby increasing blood pressure.
23. Side effects to expect with ACE inhibitors include nausea, fatigue, headache, diarrhea, and orthostatic hypotension. Side effects to report include swelling face, eyes, lips, dyspnea, neutropenia, nephrotoxicity, hyperkalemia, chronic cough, and the development of pregnancy.
24. Angiotensin II receptor inhibitors block the angiotensin II from binding to receptor sites in vascular smooth muscle and the adrenal gland. This prevents elevation of pressure and sodium-retaining properties of angiotensin II.
25. Side effects to expect with alpha$_1$ adrenergic blockers include drowsiness, headache, dizziness, weakness, tachycardia, and fainting.

Copyright © 2001 by Mosby, Inc. All rights reserved.

27. What is the anticipated side effect seen with minoxidil (Loniten, Minodyl)?

28. To what drug classification does guanadrel (Hylorel) belong?

29. What is the ending of generic drug names belonging to the classification ACE inhibitors?

30. What is the ending of generic drug names belonging to the classification angiotensin II receptor antagonists?

31. What is the ending of generic drug names belonging to the classification calcium ion antagonists?

32. What is the ending of generic drug names belonging to the classification alpha$_1$ adrenergic blocking agents?

26. Sudden discontinuation of centrally acting alpha$_2$ agonists can produce a rebound effect with sudden increase in blood pressure.

27. The anticipated side effect seen with minoxidil is hair growth on body.

28. Guanadrel is a peripheral acting adrenergic antagonist.

29. Generic drug names of ACE inhibitors end in "-pril" (enalapril, captopril, etc.).

30. Generic drug names of angiotensin II receptor antagonists end in "-sartan" (e.g., candesartan, losartan).

31. Generic drug names of calcium ion antagonists end in "-pine", except for diltiazem and verapamil.

32. Generic drug names of alpha$_1$ adrenergic blocking agents end in "-azosin".

Copyright © 2001 by Mosby, Inc.   All rights reserved.

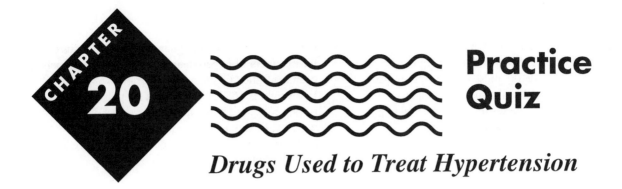

CHAPTER 20

Practice Quiz

Drugs Used to Treat Hypertension

COMPLETION

Complete the following statements.

1. _____ pressure is the difference between the systolic and diastolic pressure.
2. The ultimate goal of antihypertensive therapy is a decrease in blood pressure through reduction in _____.
3. Smoking causes _____ of blood vessels and results in_____.
4. What classes of diuretics can cause hypokalemia?
5. Why must diabetic patients be monitored closely while on beta-adrenergic blocking agents?
6. What symptoms may develop during initiation of therapy with ACE inhibitors?
7. What classification of antihypertensive agents may cause a persistent dry cough?
8. Why shouldn't patients who suspect they may be pregnant receive angiotensin II receptor antagonists?
9. What effect do calcium ion antagonists have on the smooth muscles of the blood vessels?
10. In what classification of antihypertensives do all generic names end in "-pril"?
11. In what classification of antihypertensives do all generic names end in "-sartan"?

ESSAY

12. Explain lifestyle changes that can help to reduce blood pressure.
13. Explain patient education that should be done during drug treatment of hypertension.

COMPUTATION

14. On admission, A.S.'s doctor orders start an IV of 1000 ml lactated Ringer's solution to run at 60 ml/hour. Using a microdrip administration set, how many gtt/min will be infused?

END-OF-CHAPTER MATH REVIEW

1. Ordered: Clonidine hydrochloride (Catapres) 0.6 mg daily in two divided doses.
   On hand: Clonidine hydrochloride (Catapres) 0.1, 0.2 mg tablets
   Give: _____ tablets of mg, and _____ tablets of mg
   Catapres is available in 0.3 mg tablets. What nursing action would be appropriate?

2. Ordered: Methyldopa (Aldomet) 3 g daily in three divided doses.
   On hand: Methyldopa (Aldomet) 500 mg tablets
   Give: _____ tablets per dose
   What time schedule should be established for this order?

CRITICAL THINKING QUESTIONS

1. H.L. is receiving methyldopa 3 g per day. A possible nursing diagnosis is sexual dysfunction related to methyldopa therapy manifested by impotence and/or failure to ejaculate. Address the health teaching needed and how the nurse might approach this subject.
2. Discuss the essential patient education needed regarding the initiation of prazosin therapy.
3. State the nursing assessments needed to monitor therapeutic response to, and/or side effects to expect or report with, beta adrenergic blocking agents and calcium antagonists.
4. Review the beta adrenergic blocking agent information in the monograph and develop patient education objectives for a patient receiving this class of drugs for treatment of hypertension.

Copyright © 2001 by Mosby, Inc.   All rights reserved.

5. P.J. is being started on a drug regimen for hypertension that includes the use of reserpine. Initially her BP is 160/100, pulse is 64, respirations are 20/minute, weight 148 lb. She seems quiet, introspective, and contributes little information other than "yes" or "no" responses during an initial assessment. What further nursing actions would be appropriate?

6. E.S., age 56, is receiving guanethidine and a diuretic for treatment of hypertension that has not previously been controlled by other antihypertensive therapy. His weight is 168 lb, BP is 190/110, pulse is 78, and respirations are 18/minute. He has type I diabetes mellitus. Design a specific plan for nursing assessments needed for E.S. before and during his antihypertensive regimen.

Copyright © 2001 by Mosby, Inc.   All rights reserved.

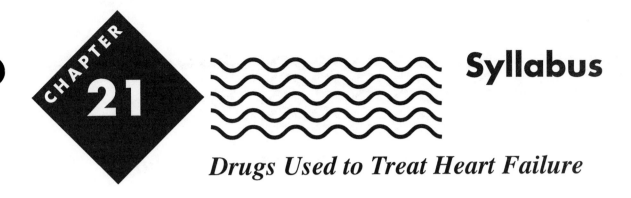

Syllabus

Drugs Used to Treat Heart Failure

CHAPTER CONTENT

Heart Failure (p. 292)
    Treatment of Heart Failure (p. 292)
    Drug Therapy for Heart Failure (p. 292)
        Drug Class: Digitalis Glycosides (p. 295)
        Drug Class: Phosphodiesterase Inhibitors (p. 298)
        Drug Class: Angiotensin Converting Enzyme
            Inhibitors (p. 300)

CHAPTER OBJECTIVES

1. Summarize the pathophysiology of heart failure including the body's compensatory mechanisms.
2. Identify the goals of treatment of heart failure.
3. Discuss the similarity in spelling of the generic names of the major cardiac glycosides.
4. Explain the process of digitalizing a patient, including the initial dose, preparation and administration of the medication, and nursing assessments needed to monitor therapeutic response and digitalis toxicity.
5. Describe safety precautions associated with the preparation and administration of digitalis glycosides.
6. State the primary actions of digitalis glycosides, angiotensin-converting enzyme inhibitors, nitrates, and calcium channel blockers on cardiac output.
7. Identify essential assessment data, nursing interventions, and health teaching needed for a patient with heart failure.

KEY WORDS

systolic dysfunction	positive inotropy
diastolic dysfunction	negative chronotrophy
inotropic agents	digitalization
digitalis toxicity	

ASSIGNMENTS

Read textbook, pp. 291-300.
Study Key Words associated with chapter content.
Study Review Sheet for Chapter 21
Complete End-of-Chapter Math Review and Critical
    Thinking Questions.

Complete Collaborative Activity as assigned by instructor.
Complete Chapter 21 Practice Quiz.
Complete Chapter 21 Exam.

COLLABORATIVE ACTIVITY

Complete the following activity. Be prepared to share your responses during in-class discussion and group work that may be assigned by the instructor.

Transcribe the following initial order to a medication administration record (MAR) and the patient Kardex. Use the MAR and Kardex records distributed by the instructor or use the records provided below.

    Gael Mazden Patient No. 123469, age 66, Dx: heart failure, Rm. 622-2, Dr. Bryce

Physician's Order Sheet:
-Meds:
    Captopril 50 mg tid
    Furosemide 120 mg po daily in the AM
    Isosorbide dinitrate 20 mg q 6 hr
    Colace 100 mg bid
-ABGs, CBC, and electrolytes, stat
-BUN, creatinine clearance, total protein, UA
-ECG stat
-O$_2$ @ 2 L/ minute via nasal cannula
-Admission weight, daily weights thereafter
-Accurate I & O; report hourly output less than 30 ml/hr
    to cardiac resident on duty (Pager # 555-1356)
-2 g sodium, soft, low-cholesterol, low-fat diet
-Oral fluids restricted to 1200 ml per 24 hours, including
    on trays
-Bedrest with BRP, HOB elevated 45° or above as
    comfortable
-Vital signs q 1 h x 12, then q 2 h, if stable
-Record neurologic status on admission and q 2 h x 24 hrs
-Skin assessment per protocol
-Alternating mattress

Copyright © 2001 by Mosby, Inc.   All rights reserved.

CHAPTER 21

Review Sheet

Drugs Used to Treat Heart Failure

The QUESTION column and the ANSWER column have been offset so that you can cover the answers while reading the questions, allowing you to assess your knowledge.

Question

1. What are the end results of systolic dysfunction of the heart?
2. What is the ultimate problem associated with diastolic dysfunction of the heart?

3. What effect does the sympathetic nervous system release of epinephrine and norepinephrine have on heart function?

4. What occurs when kidney perfusion is diminished?

5. Define the action of inotropic agents.

6. Why are diuretics used in the treatment of heart failure?

7. Name two common loop diuretics used in the treatment of heart failure.

8. List the six cardinal signs of heart disease and give a rationale for their occurrence.

Answer

1. The end result of systolic dysfunction of the heart is inability of the heart to pump with sufficient force to pump all the blood from the heart to maintain sufficient cardiac output to meet the body's oxygenation needs.
2. Due to diastolic dysfunction of the heart, residual volume remains from the previous contraction and the left ventricle does not fill adequately prior to next contraction. Back-pressure builds up in the lungs and peripheral vasculature that results in symptoms of pulmonary congestion and peripheral edema.
3. When the sympathetic nervous system releases epinephrine and norepinephrine, stimulation of the sympathetic nervous system produces tachycardia and an increase in cardiac contractility, thereby increasing cardiac output.
4. The kidney conserves sodium, which increases circulating blood volume. As this progresses there is an increase in capillary pressure and edema forms.
5. Inotropic agents increase the force of contraction of the heart as it beats, resulting in increased cardiac output to meet the body's oxygenation needs.
6. Diuretics are used in the treatment of heart failure to reduce fluid and sodium overload associated with heart failure.
7. Loop diuretics used for heart failure include furosemide (Lasix), bumetanide (Bumex), and torsemide (Demadex).

Copyright © 2001 by Mosby, Inc.   All rights reserved.

9. What classes of drugs are used to treat heart failure and what are the desired actions of each?

10. What nursing assessments should be performed at regular intervals to assess cardiac function?

11. Describe essential patient education and health promotion for patients being treated for heart failure.

12. List the nursing assessments that should be performed on a regular basis for a cardiac patient.

13. What is the desired therapeutic outcome of administering a digitalis glycoside?

14. Explain why a "loading dose" or digitalization is done.

15. Are digitoxin and digoxin interchangeable drugs?

16. List the common symptoms of digitalis toxicity.

17. What data should be gathered *before* administering a dose of a digitalis glycoside?

8. The six cardinal signs of heart disease are dyspnea, associated with inadequate tissue perfusion and diastolic dysfunction; chest pain, resulting from inadequate oxygen to support myocardium function; fatigue, due to depleted oxygen to body tissue; edema, because the left ventricle is not pumping adequate volumes of blood and a back-pressure builds up in the lungs (causing dyspnea) and the peripheral blood vessels, causing interstitial edema; syncope, due to insufficient oxygen to meet the brain's needs; and palpitations, caused by sympathetic nervous system's release of epinephrine and norepinephrine that produces tachycardia and arrhythmias.

9. The drug classes used to treat heart failure and their desired actions include vasodilator drugs, which decrease peripheral resistance the heart has to pump against; inotropic drugs, which increase force of each heart contraction resulting in increased cardiac output (CO); and diuretics, which reduce fluid volume, sodium, and peripheral resistance.

10. Mental status, vital signs (T, P, R), blood pressure, heart and lung sounds, skin color, neck vein status, presence of clubbing, CVP, abdomen size, fluid volume status, nutrition, activity and exercise tolerance, anxiety level, and laboratory tests should be checked regularly to assess cardiac function.

11. See textbook, pp. 294-295.

12. For cardiac patients, regular assessment of the respiratory rate, level of dyspnea seen in relation to exertional effort, and the degree of fatigue being experienced should be performed. Also, monitor for the occurrence of syncope and frequency of palpitations. Check for skin color, neck vein distention, pulse rate and rhythm, and blood pressure on a regularly scheduled basis. Perform auscultation and percussion of the lungs and heart. Check for the presence or absence of edema and for clubbing.

13. Digitalis glycosides slow and strengthen the heartbeat, allowing the heart to empty and fill completely, thereby improving circulation.

14. The process of digitalization allows the blood level of digitalis glycoside to be raised rapidly so the therapeutic effects can occur more rapidly. Once a therapeutic level [for digoxin (Lanoxin), 0.9 to 1.2 ng/ml] is achieved, the patient can be switched to a daily maintenance dose.

15. Digitoxin and digoxin cannot be interchanged. The onset, peak, and duration of each drug are different.

16. Common symptoms of digitalis toxicity include anorexia, nausea, extreme fatigue, weakness of arms and legs, visual disturbances, and psychiatric disturbances.

Copyright © 2001 by Mosby, Inc.   All rights reserved.

18. Under what conditions should two qualified nurses check a dose of digitalis?

19. When should a blood sample be drawn to measure the level of digitalis glycoside in the blood?

20. Why should a patient taking a digitalis glycoside be cautioned not to take an antacid within 2 hours of taking the digitalis without first consulting the physician?

21. What effect can the concurrent use of a digitalis glycoside and a diuretic have?

22. What is treatment for digitalis toxicity?

23. What is the action of phosphodiesterase inhibitors in the treatment of heart failure?

24. Name two phosphodiesterase inhibitors used to treat heart failure.

25. What is the action of ACE inhibitors in the treatment of heart failure?

17. Before administering a digitalis glycoside, apical pulse should be taken for one full minute. Consult the physician before administering the prescribed dose if the apical rate is below 60 beats per minute in an adult, or below 90 beats per minute in a child. When functioning in a nursing home environment, it may be permissible to take a radial pulse for one minute. Always check the clinical site's policies; if in doubt, take by the apical method.

18. Any time the dose requires calculation, two qualified nurses should check the dose.

19. Draw blood to measure the level of digitalis glycoside before the daily dose or at least 6–8 hours after administration of the last dose of digitalis glycoside.

20. An antacid taken with a digitalis glycoside reduces the absorption of the digitalis.

21. When taken with a digitalis glycoside, diuretics may induce hypokalemia, which may result in signs of digitalis toxicity.

22. To treat for digitalis toxicity, stop digitalis, stop potassium-depleting diuretics, and check potassium level and administer prescribed potassium if deficient. If signs of toxicity are severe and life-threatening, the antidote for digoxin, digoxin immune Fab (Digibind), may be administered.

23. Phosphodiesterase inhibitors increase the force of contraction of the myocardium, thereby increasing cardiac output (CO). They also cause relaxation of vascular smooth muscle, resulting in vasodilation that reduces preload and afterload.

24. Two phosphodiesterase inhibitors used to treat heart failure are amrinone (Inocor) and milrinone (Primacor).

25. ACE inhibitors reduce afterload by blocking angiotensin II-mediated peripheral vasoconstriction; they also reduce circulating blood volume by inhibiting aldosterone, allowing excretion of excess water.

Copyright © 2001 by Mosby, Inc. All rights reserved.

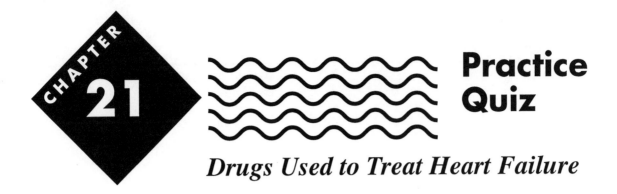

CHAPTER 21

Practice Quiz

Drugs Used to Treat Heart Failure

COMPLETION

Complete the following statements.

1. _____ is the slowing of the heart rate.
2. _____ agents increase the force of contraction of the heart as it beats.
3. _____ is another term for administering a loading dose of a digitalis glycoside.
4. The _____ pulse should be taken for _____ minute before administering a digitalis glycoside in a hospital setting.
5. Digoxin should be scheduled (before, after) meals to prevent _____.

ESSAY

6. Explain the action of digoxin.
7. Explain the actions of phosphodiesterase inhibitors and angiotensin-converting enzyme inhibitors in the treatment of heart failure.
8. Explain health teaching that should be performed for a patient being started on therapy with angiotensin-converting enzyme inhibitors.

END-OF-CHAPTER MATH REVIEW

1. T.A., age 64, weight 165 lbs, is in emergency room with stat orders:
   Ordered: Digoxin 6 mcg/Kg, IV, stat
   On hand: Digoxin 0.1 mg/ml
   165 lbs = _____ Kg
   Based on this order, how many mcg of digoxin would be given stat? _____ mcg or _____ mg

   Use any drug reference to determine the following:
   -Is digoxin given IV diluted or undiluted?
   -What rate of IV injection is recommended?
   -What IV solution(s) is digoxin compatible with?

2. T.A. is transferred from the emergency room to the coronary unit for 24 hours. The following orders exist for medications:
   Ordered: Digoxin 0.125 mg, IV q 6 hours after stat dose
   On hand: Digoxin 0.1 mg/ml and digoxin 0.25 mg/ml
   Give: Digoxin _____ ml of _____ mg/ ml
3. Following digitalization T.A. is placed on a maintenance dose as follows:
   Ordered: Digoxin 0.375 mg daily
   On hand: Digoxin 0.125 mg and 0.25 mg tablets
   Give: _____ tablets of _____ mg tablet(s)

CRITICAL THINKING QUESTIONS

1. During the digitalization process what assessments should be made on a continuum? Discuss the rationale for these observations.
2. In addition to the medications listed above, T.A. is started on furosemide 60 mg daily. What is the action of furosemide? Explain the nursing assessments that should be made to evaluate the effectiveness of the diuretic therapy.
3. Describe the purpose of drug therapy for heart failure when administering vasodilator drugs such as nitroprusside or nifedipine, a calcium channel blocker.

Copyright © 2001 by Mosby, Inc.   All rights reserved.

Syllabus

Drugs Used to Treat Arrhythmias

CHAPTER CONTENT

Arrhythmias (p. 301)
Treatment for Arrhythmias (p. 302)
Drug Therapy for Arrhythmias (p. 302)
    Antiarrhythmic Agents (p. 304)

CHAPTER OBJECTIVES

1. Describe the therapeutic response that should be observable when an antiarrhythmic agent is administered.
2. Identify baseline nursing assessments that should be implemented during the treatment of arrhythmias.
3. List the dosage forms and precautions needed in the preparation of intravenous lidocaine for the treatment of arrhythmias.
4. Cite common side effects that may be observed with the administration of amiodarone, bretylium tosylate, disopyramide, lidocaine, flecainide, mexiletine, phenytoin, procainamide, quinidine, and tocainide.
5. Identify the potential effects of muscle relaxants used during surgical intervention when combined with antiarrhythmic therapy.

KEY WORDS

electrical system
arrhythmias
atrial flutter
atrial fibrillation

paroxysmal
    supraventricular
    tachycardia
atrioventricular block
tinnitus

ASSIGNMENTS

Read textbook, pp. 301-315.
Study Key Words associated with chapter content.
Study Review Sheet for Chapter 22.
Complete End-of-Chapter Math Review and Critical Thinking Questions.
Complete Chapter 22 Practice Quiz.
Complete Chapter 22 Exam.

Copyright © 2001 by Mosby, Inc.   All rights reserved.

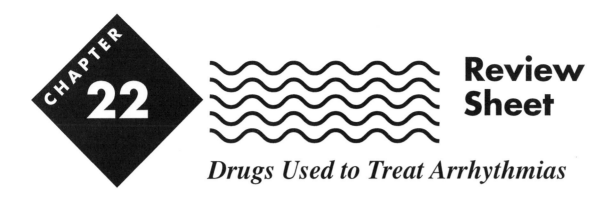

CHAPTER 22

Review Sheet

Drugs Used to Treat Arrhythmias

The QUESTION column and the ANSWER column have been offset so that you can cover the answer while reading the question, allowing you to assess your knowledge.

Question

1. Define *arrhythmia*.
2. What function does the electric system of the heart have on heart action?
3. Review the sequence of the heart's conduction system.

4. How are arrhythmias produced?

5. Define *sinus arrhythmia, sinus tachycardia, sinus bradycardia*, and *premature ventricular contraction.*

6. What is a pulse deficit?

7. What electrolyte is responsible for electrical system conduction for the SA and AV nodes?

8. What electrolyte is responsible for electrical system conduction for the atrial muscle, the His-Purkinje system, and the ventricular muscle?
9. What is the goal of treatment for arrhythmias?

10. What effect do Class I, Ia, Ib, and Ic agents have on the electrical conduction system of the heart?

Answer

1. Any heart rate or rhythm other than normal sinus rhythm is an arrhythmia.
2. The electric system of the heart sequences the muscle contractions of the heart to provide an optimal volume of blood per beat of the heart.
3. The heart's conduction system goes from SA node to AV node to Bundle of His to Purkinje fibers to ventricle muscle tissue.
4. Arrhythmias are produced by the abnormal firing of the pacemaker cells and/or the blockage of the normal electrical system pathway.
5. Sinus arrhythmia is a variable increase in heart rate originating from the SA node. The increase in rate may parallel the inspiratory phase of respirations. Sinus tachycardia is a regular rhythm of the pulse with an accelerated rate greater than 120 beats per minute. Sinus bradycardia is a regular rhythm of the pulse, but the rate is slower than 60 beats per minute. In premature ventricular contraction, the beat occurs before the regular ventricular contraction as a result of an electrical impulse arising in the ventricle outside the normal conduction pathway.
6. Pulse deficit is the difference between the apical and radial pulse rates; radial is generally lower than apical. For example: apical pulse = 74, radial pulse = 64, pulse deficit = 10.
7. Calcium ions are responsible for electrical system conduction for the SA and AV nodes.

8. Sodium is responsible for electrical system conduction for the atrial muscle, the His-Purkinje system, and the ventricular muscle.
9. The goal of treatment for arrhythmias is to restore normal sinus rhythm and maintain adequate cardiac output to maintain tissue perfusion.

Copyright © 2001 by Mosby, Inc. All rights reserved.

11. What methods are used to assess arrhythmias?

12. Review the six cardinal signs of cardiovascular disease.

13. Why can mental status/level of consciousness (LOC) be important when assessing a cardiac patient?
14. What type of changes in the vital signs should be reported to the physician?
15. Why is it important to monitor hourly urine output in a patient with arrhythmias?
16. When is the use of adenosine (Adenocard) indicated?

17. When beta-adrenergic blocking agents are administered what cardiac response can be anticipated?
18. Bretylium tosylate (Bretylol) belong to which class of antiarrhythmic agents?

19. When lidocaine (Xylocaine) is ordered for an arrhythmia, what should the nurse check on the bottle BEFORE using the medication for IV administration?
20. What agent is the drug of choice for treatment of ventricular arrhythmias associated with acute myocardial infarction and ventricular tachycardia?
21. What drug, also used for seizure disorders, may be used to treat paroxysmal atrial tachycardia and ventricular arrhythmias, particularly those induced by digitalis toxicity?
22. What action does quinidine have on the heart?

23. When should blood samples for quinidine sulfate levels be drawn in relationship to doses being administered?
24. What is cinchonism?

25. What initial assessments of the heart disorder should be performed when an arrhythmia is suspected?

26. Review assessments performed for an individual with a heart disorder and compare these with premedication assessments listed throughout this chapter.
27. Why is physical activity curtailed in a patient having arrhythmias?

10. The effects of Class I, Ia, Ib, and Ic agents are as follows: I is a myocardial depressant (inhibits sodium ion movement); Ia causes prolonged duration electrical stimulation on cells and refractory time between electrical impulses; Ib shortens duration of electrical stimulation and time interval between electrical impulses; Ic is the most potent antiarrhythmic, causing myocardial depression and slowing conduction rate through the atria and the ventricles.
11. ECG monitoring, EPS (electrophysiologic studies), exercise electrocardiography, and laboratory values are used to assess for cardiac arrhythmias.
12. The six cardinal signs of cardiac disease are dyspnea, chest pain, fatigue, edema, syncope, and palpitations.
13. Mental status/LOC indicates whether there is adequate cerebral tissue perfusion.
14. See textbook, p. 303.

15. Hourly outputs reflect whether the kidney tissues are being adequately perfused.
16. Adenosine is indicated in treatment of paroxysmal supraventricular tachycardia that involves conduction in the SA node, atrium, or AV node.
17. Reduction in heart rate, systolic blood pressure, and cardiac output result from use of beta-adrenergic blocking agents.
18. Bretylium tosylate is an adrenergic blocking agent, class III antiarrhythmic agent.

19. The bottle must be labeled "Xylocaine for Arrhythmia" or "Lidocaine Without Preservatives."

20. Lidocaine (Xylocaine) is the drug of choice.

21. Phenytoin may be used to treat some cardiac arrhythmias, as well as seizure disorders.
22. Quinidine stabilizes the rate of conduction resulting in a slow, regular pulse rate.

23. Blood samples for quinidine sulfate levels should be drawn before the daily dose or at least 6 hours after administration.
24. The signs and symptoms associated with quinidine toxicity (known as cinchonism) include salivation, tinnitus, headache, visual disturbances, and mental confusion.
25. Electrocardiogram should be performed when an arrhythmia is suspected.

26. See textbook, pp. 303-304, and see individual monographs throughout the chapter.

Copyright © 2001 by Mosby, Inc. All rights reserved.

28. Why is O_2 administration required prn when an arrhythmia occurs?

29. What are the drawbacks of using amiodarone hydrochloride (Cordarone)?

27. To conserve oxygen use so that the available oxygen can be used to meet the body's basic needs, physical activity is curtailed in patients with arrhythmias. Reduced oxygen levels (hypoxia) induce arrhythmias.

28. To prevent hypoxia and the development of arrhythmias, O_2 is administered prn.

29. Amiodarone hydrochloride requires hospitalization during loading dose and maintenance dose is difficult to establish. Life-threatening arrhythmias may recur at unpredictable intervals. Once the drug is used, switching to a different antiarrhythmic is difficult because the body may store the drug; therefore, a drug interaction with the newly prescribed antiarrhythmic may occur.

Copyright © 2001 by Mosby, Inc. All rights reserved.

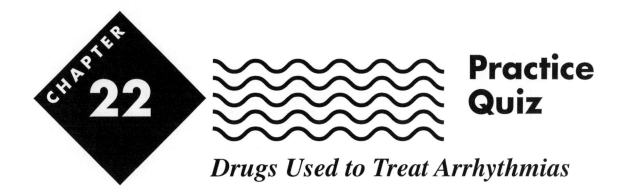

COMPLETION

Complete the following statements.

The therapeutic goals of antiarrhythmic therapy are:

1. _____

2. _____

3. _____

4. Basic mental status functioning may be impaired with insufficient cardiac output as a result of _____.

5. The action of Class I antiarrhythmic agents is:

6. The action of Class Ia antiarrhythmic agents is _____.

The actions of beta adrenergic blocking agents are:

7. _____

8. _____

9. _____

10. Why should the label on a lidocaine container used for arrhythmias be different from the lidocaine used as a local anesthetic agent?

11. Cinchonism is _____.

12. State the sequence of the heart's conduction system.

13. The initial assessment for a suspected arrhythmia is _____.

List the six cardinal signs of heart disease that should be monitored on a continuum whenever a heart disorder is suspected.

14. _____

15. _____

16. _____

17. _____

18. _____

19. _____

END-OF-CHAPTER MATH REVIEW

1. Ordered: Quinidine 0.8 grams, po, tid.
   On hand: Quinidine 200 mg tablets
   Give: _____ tablets per dose
   Give: _____ total grams in 24 hours

2. Ordered: Procainamide hydrochloride (Pronestyl) 1 g q 6 h.
   On hand: Procainamide hydrochloride (Pronestyl) 250 mg capsules
   Give: _____ capsules per dose

CRITICAL THINKING QUESTIONS

Situation: Adenosine (Adenocard) 6 mg IV bolus was given stat to a patient in the emergency room being treated for paroxysmal supraventricular tachycardia. At post conference the instructor discusses this case with the student nurses.

Answer the following questions using any reference books:

1. What is paroxysmal supraventricular tachycardia and why is this dangerous to the patient?

2. What is the normal conduction of impulses through the heart?

Copyright © 2001 by Mosby, Inc.   All rights reserved.

3. Look up the following information for the drug adenosine:
   Drug action:
   Dosage:
   Preparation of drug for IV use:
   Dilution: Yes   No
   Solutions that can be used to dilute the IV medication:
   Rate of administration:
   Incompatibility:
   Side effects to expect:

Situation: Doctor's order: Quinidine sulfate 200 mg, po, qid.

1. What time schedule would be used to fulfill this order? When a quinidine serum level is ordered, based on the time schedule established, when would the laboratory draw the blood sample?

2. What nursing assessments should be made during the administration of quinidine sulfate? What health teaching should be done?

Situation: The doctor orders disopyramide (Norpace) 150 mg, q 6 h.

1. What time schedule would be used to administer the drug?

2. After a week of therapy the therapeutic blood level report from the laboratory is 8 mg/L. What nursing action(s) would be initiated?

Copyright © 2001 by Mosby, Inc.   All rights reserved.

CHAPTER 23

Drugs Used to Treat Angina Pectoris

CHAPTER CONTENT

Angina Pectoris (p. 316)
Treatment of Angina Pectoris (p. 316)
Drug Therapy for Angina Pectoris (p. 318)
    Drug Class: Nitrates (p. 318)
    Drug Class: Beta Adrenergic Blocking Agents
       (p. 321)
    Drug Class: Calcium Ion Antagonists (p. 321)

CHAPTER OBJECTIVES

1. Describe the actions of nitrates, beta adrenergic
   blockers, and calcium channel blockers on the
   myocardial tissue of the heart.
2. Identify assessment data needed to evaluate an
   anginal attack.
3. Implement medication therapy health teaching to an
   anginal patient in the clinical setting.

KEY WORDS

angina pectoris
ischemic heart disease
chronic stable angina
unstable angina
variant angina

ASSIGNMENTS

Read textbook, pp. 316-323.
Study Key Words associated with chapter content.
Study Review Sheet for Chapter 23
Complete End-of-Chapter Math Review and Critical
    Thinking Questions.
Complete Collaborative Activity as assigned by instructor.
Complete Chapter 23 Practice Quiz
Complete Chapter 23 Exam.

COLLABORATIVE ACTIVITIES

Prepare a teaching plan for an individual who has
nitroglycerin sublingual prn, and nifedipine (Procardia),
30 mg sustained-release capsules once daily.

Copyright © 2001 by Mosby, Inc.   All rights reserved.

Review Sheet

Drugs Used to Treat Angina Pectoris

The QUESTION column and the ANSWER column have been offset so that you can cover the answer while reading the questions, allowing you to assess your knowledge.

Question	Answer
1. Explain the underlying cause of anginal pain.	
2. Review the various presenting symptoms of angina.	1. The pain and discomfort of angina is caused by the lack of an adequate oxygen supply to the cells in the heart (ischemic heart disease). The underlying etiology is atherosclerosis or spasms of the coronary arteries.
3. Compare the precipitating factors associated with chronic stable angina, unstable angina, and variant angina.	2. See textbook, p. 316.
4. What are the desired therapeutic outcomes during treatment of angina?	3. Chronic stable angina is precipitated by physical exertion or stress. Unstable angina is precipitated by unpredictable factors such as atherosclerotic narrowing, vasospasm, or thrombus formation. Variant angina occurs at rest. The underlying etiology is vasospasm of a coronary artery that reduces blood flow through the coronary arteries to the heart tissue.
5. What questions should be asked during a nursing assessment related to an angina attack?	4. The desired therapeutic outcomes of treatment for angina are decreased frequency and severity of anginal attacks, increased tolerance to activities, and increased quality of life. Pharmacologic treatment of angina is to reduce oxygen demand by lowering heart rate, myocardial contractility, and ventricular volume.
6. What are the actions of nitrates, beta-adrenergic blockers, and calcium channel blockers on the myocardial tissue of the heart? Name two examples of each drug class used to treat angina pectoris.	5. See textbook, p. 317.
7. What is the drug of choice for acute attacks of angina pectoris?	6. Nitrates do not increase total coronary artery blood flow. They cause relaxation of peripheral vascular smooth muscle that results in dilation of arteries and veins, reducing preload and leading to decreased oxygen demands on the heart. They do not dilate large coronary arteries and redistribute blood flow within the heart. Beta-adrenergic blocking agents decrease myocardial oxygen demands by blocking beta adrenergic receptors in the heart, reducing stimulation by

Copyright © 2001 by Mosby, Inc. All rights reserved.

norepinephrine and epinephrine, which normally increases heart rate. Beta blockers also reduce blood pressure.

Calcium channel blockers decrease myocardial oxygen demands and increase myocardial blood supply by coronary artery dilation. These agents block movement of calcium ions across the cell membrane, resulting in 1) inhibition of smooth muscle contraction; 2) dilation of blood vessels, including coronary arteries; and 3) decreased resistance to blood flow as a result of dilation of peripheral vessels.

Select two drugs from each classification from Tables 11-3, 23-1, and 23-2 in textbook.

8. Why is it important to teach patients taking nitroglycerin not to use alcohol?

9. What dose forms are available for nitroglycerin?

10. What side effects can be expected when amyl nitrite medications are used?

11. What premedication assessments should be performed prior to therapy with nitrates?

12. Describe the procedure for administering nitroglycerin sublingually, via translingual spray, topical ointment, transmucosal tablets, and topical disk.

13. How does one evaluate anginal attacks and what health teaching is needed for an individual who has anginal attacks?

14. What are some guidelines used during the preparation and administration of IV nitroglycerin?

15. What are the desired therapeutic outcomes of the use of beta blocker therapy for treatment of anginal pain?

16. What premedication assessments should be performed prior to administering beta blockers?

17. What is the desired result of the use of calcium ion antagonists to treat angina?

7. Nitroglycerin, administered sublingually, is the drug of choice for acute attacks of angina pectoris.

8. Alcohol use results in vasodilation and may lead to postural hypotension.

9. Sublingual tablets, transmucosal tablets, translingual spray, topical disks, sustained-release capsules, topical ointment, and intravenous forms of nitroglycerin are available.

10. Headache and hypotension caused by the vasodilation of blood vessels are side effects of amyl nitrate treatment.

11. Assess for pain level, location, duration, intensity, and pattern, and obtain history of most recent nitrate use before beginning amyl nitrate therapy.

12. Procedure for administration of the various forms of nitroglycerin: Textbook, Chapter 10, Percutaneous Administration, and Chapter 23, pp. 319-320.

13. See textbook, pp. 317-318.

14. See textbook, p. 321.

15. The desired therapeutic outcomes of beta blocker therapy are decreased frequency and severity of anginal attacks, increased tolerance of activities, and decreased use of nitroglycerin for acute anginal attacks.

16. Before administering beta blockers, take BP in supine and standing position, check for history of respiratory disorders such as COPD, and check for history of diabetes. If patient is a diabetic see if the physician wants baseline serum glucose studies before initiating the medication.

17. The desired action of calcium ion antagonists in the treatment of angina is decreased myocardial oxygen demands by increasing myocardial blood supply via coronary arteries and decreased resistance to blood flow and dilate peripheral vessels, resulting in decreased workload of the heart.

Copyright © 2001 by Mosby, Inc. All rights reserved.

Practice Quiz

Drugs Used to Treat Angina Pectoris

ESSAY

1. List a minimum of four symptoms of an angina attack.
2. What nursing assessments are appropriate for an individual who arrives at the emergency room complaining of chest pain? What if the person has a history of angina pectoris?
3. Explain the lifestyle modifications needed as part of the treatment of angina pectoris.
4. How often should sublingual nitrates be administered when ordered prn?
5. How often are sustained-release tablets of nitroglycerin administered?
6. How are transmucosal tablets administered and how often is this form of a nitrate administered daily?
7. State the procedure for administering translingual nitrate spray, topical ointment, and transdermal disks.
8. State the mechanism of action of nitrates, calcium channel blockers, and beta adrenergic agents in the treatment of anginal pain.
9. Name two calcium channel blockers and two beta adrenergic blockers used to treat angina.
10. Explain the premedication assessments that should be performed before administering nitrates, beta blockers, and calcium channel blockers.

END-OF-CHAPTER MATH REVIEW

1. Ordered: Nitroglycerin 0.3 mg, SL, prn for chest pain
   On hand: Nitroglycerin 0.15 mg SL tablets.
   Give: _____ tablets
2. Ordered: Nifedipine (Procardia) 10 mg, SL for acute pain
   On hand: Nifedipine (Procardia) 10 mg capsules
   Give: _____ capsules
   Explain the procedure for sublingual administration of the nifedipine.

3. Ordered: Propranolol hydrochloride (Inderal), 160 mg, qd
   On hand: Propranolol hydrochloride (Inderal) concentrated oral solution 80 mg/ml
   Give: _____ ml.

CRITICAL THINKING QUESTIONS

Situation: P.S., a 64-year-old male, comes to the emergency room with acute chest pain. He is holding his chest with his fist directly over the sternum. He appears diaphoretic. He is in work clothes and has been mowing the lawn. It is 98 °F outside.

1. What nursing actions would be appropriate immediately?
2. What drug(s) would likely be ordered if this is acute angina pectoris?
3. Describe the correct procedure for administering nitroglycerin SL.
4. If a stat dose of nitroglycerin sublingual spray is ordered, explain how you would instruct the patient to give it.
5. When giving A.M. medications in the nursing home, the nurse comes to an order to apply Nitro-Dur patch 2.5 mg. The MAR (medication administration record) indicates the prior patch was applied to the right scapula area. The patch is not there. How would you proceed to execute the order?

 Copyright © 2001 by Mosby, Inc.   All rights reserved.

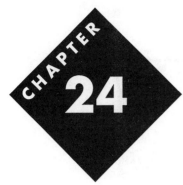

CHAPTER 24

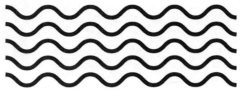

Syllabus

Drugs Used to Treat Peripheral Vascular Disease

CHAPTER CONTENTS

CHAPTER OBJECTIVES

1. List the baseline assessments used to evaluate a patient with peripheral vascular disease (PVD).
2. Identify specific measures the patient can use to improve peripheral circulation and prevent complications from peripheral vascular disease.
3. Identify the systemic effects to expect when peripheral vasodilators are administered.
4. Explain why hypotension and tachycardia occur frequently with the use of peripheral vasodilators.
5. Develop measurable objectives for patient education for patients with peripheral vascular disease.
6. State both pharmacologic and nonpharmacologic goals of treatment for peripheral vascular disease.

KEY WORDS

arteriosclerosis obliterans
intermittent claudication
paresthesias
Raynaud's disease
vasospasm

ASSIGNMENTS

Read textbook, pp. 324-331.
Study Key Words associated with chapter content.
Study Review Sheet for Chapter 24.
Complete End-of-Chapter Math Review and Critical Thinking Questions.
Complete Chapter 24 Exam.

Copyright © 2001 by Mosby, Inc.   All rights reserved.

CHAPTER **24**

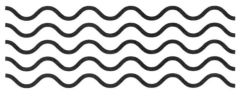

Review Sheet

Drugs Used to Treat Peripheral Vascular Disease

The QUESTION column and the ANSWER column have been offset so that you can cover the answer before reading the questions, thus allowing you to assess your knowledge.

Question	Answer
1. Explain the pathophysiology of intermittent claudication, vasospasm, paresthesia, arteriosclerosis obliterans, and Raynaud's disease.	
2. What are the goals of treatment of arteriosclerosis obliterans?	1. See textbook, p. 324.
3. What actions can be taken by a patient with Raynaud's disease to reduce or stop vasospastic attacks?	2. Improve blood flow, relieve pain, and prevent skin ulcerations and/or gangrene.
4. What nursing assessments should be made on a regular basis when peripheral vasodilators are prescribed?	3. Avoid cold temperature, emotional stress, tobacco, and drugs known to induce attacks.
5. Describe the health teaching needed when peripheral vascular disease (PVD) is diagnosed that would promote improved tissue perfusion.	4. Assess for color and temperature of the hands, fingers, legs, and feet. Check for signs and symptoms of skin breakdown, presence of limb pain, or a reduction in sensation in the extremities. Pedal pulses and radial pulse rates should be taken and recorded q 4 h during hospitalization and bid upon discharge.

1. Explain the pathophysiology of intermittent claudication, vasospasm, paresthesia, arteriosclerosis obliterans, and Raynaud's disease.
2. What are the goals of treatment of arteriosclerosis obliterans?
3. What actions can be taken by a patient with Raynaud's disease to reduce or stop vasospastic attacks?
4. What nursing assessments should be made on a regular basis when peripheral vasodilators are prescribed?
5. Describe the health teaching needed when peripheral vascular disease (PVD) is diagnosed that would promote improved tissue perfusion.

6. What is the action of pentoxifylline (Trental) and cilostazol (Pletal)?
7. What type of vascular conditions may be treated using peripheral vasodilating agents?

8. What is the mechanism of action of vasodilators used to treat PVD?

9. What are the side effects to expect with the administration of vasodilating agents?

Answer

1. See textbook, p. 324.

2. Improve blood flow, relieve pain, and prevent skin ulcerations and/or gangrene.

3. Avoid cold temperature, emotional stress, tobacco, and drugs known to induce attacks.

4. Assess for color and temperature of the hands, fingers, legs, and feet. Check for signs and symptoms of skin breakdown, presence of limb pain, or a reduction in sensation in the extremities. Pedal pulses and radial pulse rates should be taken and recorded q 4 h during hospitalization and bid upon discharge.

5. See textbook, pp. 326-327.

6. Trental increases RBC (red blood cell) flexibility, decreases concentration of fibrinogen in the blood, and prevents aggregation of RBCs and platelets, thus preventing blood clotting. Cilostazol inhibits platelet aggregation and promotes vasodilation.

7. Intermittent claudication, arteriosclerosis obliterans, vasospasms associated with thrombophlebitis, nocturnal leg cramps, and Raynaud's disease.

8. Relaxation of peripheral arterial blood vessels, thereby increasing blood flow to the extremities.

9. Flushing, tingling, sweating. May also produce orthostatic hypotension and tachycardia. Also may cause possible nervousness and weakness as therapy progresses.

Copyright © 2001 by Mosby, Inc. All rights reserved.

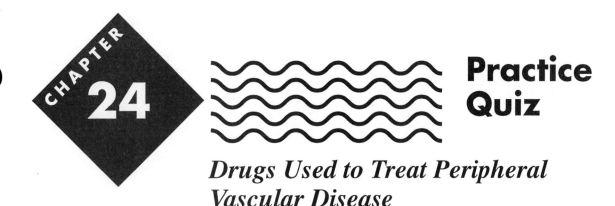

CHAPTER 24

Practice Quiz

Drugs Used to Treat Peripheral Vascular Disease

ESSAY

1. Explain why hemorrheologic agents and vasodilators may relieve the symptoms of peripheral vascular disease (PVD).
2. What nonpharmacologic measures can improve peripheral circulation?
3. Explain how to assess tissue that is affected by PVD.
4. What is the desired therapeutic outcome to expect from the use of vasodilators to treat PVD?

END-OF-CHAPTER MATH REVIEW

1. Ordered: Cyclandelate (Cyclospasmol) 200 mg qid x 4 days, then 400 mg/day bid
   On hand: Cyclandelate (Cyclospasmol) 200 mg and 400 mg tablets
   How many 200 mg tablets would be needed to administer the first 4 days of dosages? _____
   How many 400 mg tablets would be needed to administer the next 5 days of dosages? _____
2. Ordered: Papaverine hydrochloride (Pavebid) 300 mg, q 12 h
   On hand: Papaverine hydrochloride (Pavebid) 150 mg time-release capsules
   Give: _____ capsules per dose

CRITICAL THINKING QUESTIONS

Situation: Mrs. Dunbar tells you when she and her husband go for their daily walks he can only go two blocks and then has to sit down because of pain in the calves of his legs. They rest a while, walk another two blocks, and the pain is back. She asks your advice.
1. What would you tell her?

Two days later, Mr. Dunbar is assigned to you for nursing care. His primary nursing diagnosis is altered tissue perfusion related to insufficient oxygenation of the lower limbs manifested by pain on walking two blocks, diminished popliteal pulses, bilaterally.
2. What nursing assessments would you plan to make?

3. What health teaching would be needed in relation to his drug therapy? He has phenoxybenzamine hydrochloride (Dibenzyline) 10 mg capsule daily ordered. Review the drug monograph and discuss the drug's action and side effects to anticipate.

Situation: Mr. Canterbury, age 76, has been suffering from arteriosclerosis obliterans with intermittent claudication. He refuses to give up smoking. At his last office visit, a prescription for Trental 400 mg tid, po with meals was written. On the way out of the exam room, he tells you, the office nurse, that the physician did not explain how this would work to improve his "leg pain."

Give him a simple explanation of what is thought to be the mechanism of action and draw a diagram that depicts "erythrocyte flexibility" and use the visual aid to assist him to understand how the drug could improve his "leg pain."

A week later, Mr. Canterbury calls the office: "That new medication you gave me for my leg pain isn't working."
1. How should you respond?

Copyright © 2001 by Mosby, Inc. All rights reserved.

CHAPTER CONTENTS

CHAPTER OBJECTIVES

1. Cite nursing assessments used to evaluate a patient's state of hydration.
2. Review possible underlying pathology that may contribute to the development of excess fluid volume in the body.
3. State which electrolytes may be altered by diuretic therapy.
4. Cite nursing assessments used to evaluate renal function.
5. Identify the effects of diuretics on blood pressure, electrolytes, and diabetic or prediabetic patients.
6. Review the signs and symptoms of electrolyte imbalance and normal laboratory values of potassium, sodium, and chloride.
7. Identify the action of diuretics.
8. Explain the rationale for administering diuretics cautiously to older patients and people with impaired renal function, cirrhosis of the liver, or diabetes mellitus.
9. Describe the goal of administering diuretics to treat hypertension, heart failure, increased intraocular pressure, or before vascular surgery in the brain.
10. List side effects that can be anticipated whenever a diuretic is administered.
11. Cite alterations in diet that may be prescribed concurrently with loop, thiazide, or potassium-sparing diuretic therapy.
12. State the nursing assessments needed to monitor therapeutic response or development of side effects to expect or report from diuretic therapy.
13. Develop objectives for patient education for patients taking loop, thiazide, and potassium-sparing diuretics.

KEY WORDS

aldosterone	orthostatic hypotension
tubule	electrolyte imbalance
Loop of Henle	hyperuricemia

ASSIGNMENTS

Read textbook pp. 332-345.
Study Key Words associated with chapter content.
Study Review Sheet for Chapter 25.
Complete End-of-Chapter Math Review and Critical
    Thinking Questions.
Complete Collaborative Activity as assigned by instructor.
Complete Chapter 25 Practice Quiz.
Complete Chapter 25 Exam.

COLLABORATIVE ACTIVITY

Complete the following as preparation for in-class discussion and group work that may be assigned by the instructor.

The doctor orders furosemide 40 mg IV stat. Refer to the drug monograph and any other drug resources necessary, then explain how the nurse would prepare and administer the dose via a saline lock that is in place. Explain how to calculate the rate of administration when the drug is given IV push.

    If administering a stat dose of furosemide (Lasix) to a patient with a Foley catheter, why should the nurse empty the catheter bag and record the amount of urine in the bag immediately before administering the stat dose of medication?

Copyright © 2001 by Mosby, Inc.   All rights reserved.

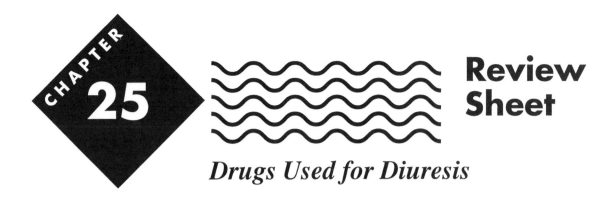

Drugs Used for Diuresis

The QUESTION column and the ANSWER column have been offset so you can cover the answer while reading the question, allowing you to assess your knowledge.

Question

1. Explain the therapeutic outcomes associated with diuretic therapy.
2. What laboratory tests should be checked to determine if kidney function is impaired?

3. What laboratory studies should be checked whenever a diuretic is prescribed?

4. What patient assessments should be performed on a regular basis when diuretics are being taken?
5. What is the action of a diuretic?

6. What are the six classes of diuretics?

7. Which class of diuretic has the most rapid onset of action? (List the four drugs.) What three routes of administration can be used for loop diuretics?

8. After administration of a loop diuretic using each of these routes, how soon will diuresis occur and how long will it last?

9. When would loop diuretics be prescribed?

10. Of the four loop diuretics, which is most frequently prescribed?
11. Would thiazide or loop diuretics be used when renal function is impaired?

Answer

1. The therapeutic outcomes of diuretic therapy are diuresis with reduction of edema and improvement in the symptoms of fluid overload and reduced blood pressure.
2. Check for elevated BUN and serum creatinine, decreased creatinine clearance, decreased urine output, and increasing edema.
3. Check Hct, serum electrolytes, blood glucose, uric acid, BUN, and serum creatinine.
4. Assess intake and output of fluids, state of hydration, presence of edema, heart rate and rhythm, blood pressure bid or qid, and daily weights. Check for signs and symptoms of electrolyte imbalance, gastric irritation, rash, hyperuricemia, and hyperglycemia. Monitor for drug interactions (e.g., digitalis glycosides, corticosteroids, lithium).
5. Diuretics inhibit the reabsorption of sodium, increasing the loss of water.
6. The six classes of diuretic are thiazide, loop, potassium-sparing, osmotic, methylxanthine, and carbonic anhydrase inhibitors. Thiazides and potassium-sparing diuretics are also available as combination products.
7. Loop diuretics are furosemide (Lasix), ethacrynic acid (Edecrin), bumetanide (Bumex), and torsemide (Demadex). Oral (po), intramuscular (IM), or intravenous (IV) routes.
8. Oral: onset, 30 to 60 minutes; peak, 1 to 2 hours; duration, 6 to 8 hours. IM: onset, 30 to 40 minutes; peak, 1 to 2 hours; duration, 5 to 6 hours. IV: onset, 5 minutes; peak 15 to 45 minutes; duration, 2 hours.
9. When rapid diuresis is needed (e.g., in pulmonary edema) or when renal function is diminished.
10. Furosemide

Copyright © 2001 by Mosby, Inc. All rights reserved.

12. What classes of diuretics can cause a loss of serum potassium (hypokalemia)?

13. What class(es) of diuretic(s) can cause an increase in serum potassium (hyperkalemia)?

14. What type(s) of diuretic(s) are used to reduce intraocular and intracranial pressure?

15. Why would a potassium-sparing and another type of diuretic be prescribed simultaneously?

16. What actions can be taken to prevent and/or treat hypokalemia?

17. What actions can be taken to prevent hyperkalemia when potassium-sparing diuretics are prescribed?

18. Are diuretics useful for edema that occurs during pregnancy?

19. What medicine may need to be ordered for patients who have gouty arthritis who require diuretics?

20. Which type of diuretic has been associated with hearing loss when used in high doses?

21. What class of antibiotics can cause hearing loss and, if combined with loop diuretics, may increase the possibility of ototoxicity?

22. After reading that diuretics can interact with digitalis glycosides to produce digitalis toxicity, what signs and symptoms would you monitor when therapy is combined?

23. What are the normal values for sodium, potassium, and chloride?

24. List six foods that are good sources of potassium.

25. Why should salicylates not be taken with furosemide for prolonged periods?

26. Describe the signs and symptoms of salicylate toxicity.

27. Which class of diuretics can affect the male libido?

28. Why are potassium-sparing diuretics not used in patients with renal failure?

29. What are the signs and symptoms of circulatory overload?

30. Why must the IV site be checked frequently when osmotic agents are administered IV?

31. How do carbonic anhydrase inhibitors decrease intraocular pressure?

32. What premedication assessments should be made before administering any type of diuretic?

11. Loop diuretics are more effective than other classes of diuretics when renal function is impaired (decreased creatinine clearance).

12. Thiazide, loop, and osmotic diuretics

13. Potassium-sparing diuretics

14. Osmotic diuretics

15. To prevent hypokalemia, improve diuresis, and lower blood pressure.

16. Give potassium supplements and/or increase dietary intake of foods rich in potassium.

17. Do not use salt substitutes that contain potassium. Maintain an adequate fluid intake. Do not administer potassium supplements.

18. Diuretics are rarely used for edema associated with pregnancy. Diuretics cross the placental barrier and may be harmful to the fetus. Consult a physician before taking any medication during pregnancy or while breastfeeding.

19. Allopurinol

20. Loop diuretics

21. Aminoglycosides: gentamicin, tobramycin, kanamycin, amikacin, neomycin, streptomycin, netilmicin.

22. Anorexia, nausea, fatigue, blurred or colored vision, bradycardia, arrhythmias.

23. Sodium: 135 to 145 mEq/L; potassium: 3.5 to 5.0 mEq/L; chloride: 95 to 110 mEq/L

24. Dried almonds; apricots, raw; avocados, raw; bananas, raw; beans, lima (cooked, boiled); carrots, raw; cocoa, plain; potatoes (cooked, boiled)

25. The potential for salicylate toxicity may be increased if taken concurrently for several days.

26. Nausea, tinnitus, fever, sweating, dizziness, mental confusion, lethargy, and impaired hearing.

27. Potassium-sparing diuretics [e.g., amiloride (Midamor), spironolactone (Aldactone)].

28. They are usually not effective as diuretics in moderate to severe renal failure and may cause hyperkalemia.

29. Bounding, full pulse; jugular vein distention; dyspnea; frothy sputum; cough.

30. If the drug leaks into tissue surrounding the blood vessel (infiltration, extravasation) it can cause tissue necrosis.

31. Carbonic anhydrase inhibitors decrease production of aqueous humor; thus are used to treat both closed-angle and open-angle glaucoma.

Copyright © 2001 by Mosby, Inc. All rights reserved.

32. Baseline vital signs, lung sounds, weight, assessment of degree of edema, level of consciousness (LOC), muscle strength, tremors, general appearance; blood glucose levels for patients with diabetes. Baseline laboratory studies as prescribed by physician.

CRITICAL THINKING QUESTIONS

1. The physician orders furosemide 80 mg stat IV push. The drug resource book states, "The rate of administration should not exceed 4 mg per minute." Based on this information, how long would it take to administer the furosemide? What other facts should be checked prior to initiating IV push of the drug?

2. R.J. is being treated for hypertension with diuretic therapy. She calls the physician's office to report she is feeling weak, light-headed, and fatigued. What additional information would be useful prior to discussing her symptoms with the physician?

Copyright © 2001 by Mosby, Inc.   All rights reserved.

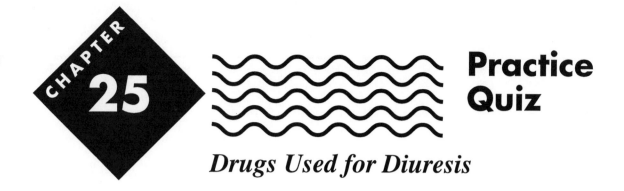

Drugs Used for Diuresis

COMPLETION

Complete the following statements.

Two major diseases treated with diuretics are:

1. _____

2. _____

List four laboratory tests used to assess the state of hydration:

3. _____

4. _____

5. _____

6. _____

The normal range for the following electrolytes is:

7. Sodium (Na^+) = _____ mEq/L

8. Potassium (K^+) = _____ mEq/L

9. The most frequently used loop diuretic is

_____.

10. Ototoxicity may occur with high doses of

_____.

11. Diabetic patients using diuretic(s) must be checked regularly for _____.

12. _____ occurs with diuretics that inhibit the excretion of uric acid.

13. _____ can occur with diuretic therapy due to reduction in total circulating fluid volume.

Name three loop diuretics.

14. _____

15. _____

16. _____

Name three thiazide diuretics.

17. _____

18. _____

19. _____

Name one potassium-sparing diuretic.

20. _____

ESSAY

21. Why is it important to know a patient's vital signs, mental status, and general appearance before administering a diuretic?

22. What action can diuretics have on uric acid in the body?

23. Which electrolytes are most commonly affected by diuretic therapy?

24. Why can the administration of a diuretic sometimes cause digitalis toxicity?

25. What antibiotics, given concurrently with diuretics, may cause ototoxicity?

26. What drug classification do each of the following diuretics belong to?
    a. furosemide
    b. torsemide
    c. hydrochlorothiazide
    d. spironolactone

27. Why are combination diuretic products used?

END-OF-CHAPTER MATH REVIEW

1. Ordered: Ethacrynic acid 50 mg IV in 50 ml 5% dextrose and water. The patient has an IV pump running that is calibrated in ml/hr. Infuse the medication over 30 minutes.
   Set the pump at _____ml/hr.

2. Ordered: Furosemide 40 mg po stat
   On hand: Furosemide 20 mg tablets
   Give: _____ tablet(s)

Copyright © 2001 by Mosby, Inc.   All rights reserved.

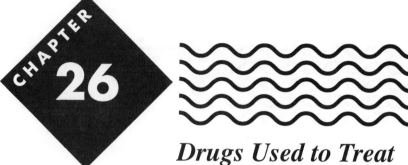

CHAPTER 26

Syllabus

Drugs Used to Treat Thromboembolic Disorders

CHAPTER CONTENTS

CHAPTER OBJECTIVES

1. State the primary purposes of anticoagulant therapy.
2. Analyze Figure 26-1 to identify the site of action of warfarin, heparin, and fibrinolytic medicine.
3. Identify the effects of anticoagulant therapy on existing blood clots.
4. Describe conditions that place an individual at risk for developing blood clots.
5. Identify specific nursing interventions that can prevent clot formation.
6. Explain laboratory data used to establish dosing of anticoagulant medications.
7. Describe specific monitoring procedures to detect hemorrhage in the anticoagulated patient.
8. Describe procedures used to ensure that the correct dose of an anticoagulant is prepared and administered.
9. Explain the specific procedures and techniques used to administer heparin subcutaneously, via intermittent administration through a heparin lock, and via intravenous infusion.
10. Identify the purpose, dosing determination, and scheduling factors associated with the use of protamine sulfate.
11. State the nursing assessments needed to monitor therapeutic response and the development of side effects to expect or report from anticoagulant therapy.
12. Develop objectives for patient education for patients receiving anticoagulant therapy.

KEY WORDS

thromboembolic diseases	extrinsic clotting pathway
thrombosis	platelet inhibitors
thrombus	anticoagulants
embolus	thrombolytic agents
intrinsic clotting pathway	fibrinolytic agents

ASSIGNMENTS

Read textbook pp. 346-358.
Study Key Words associated with chapter content.
Complete and study Review Sheet for Chapter 26.
Complete End-of-Chapter Math Review and Critical Thinking Questions.
Complete Chapter 26 Practice Quiz.
Complete Chapter 26 Exam.

Copyright © 2001 by Mosby, Inc.   All rights reserved.

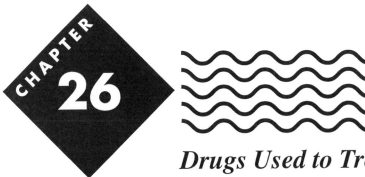

Review Sheet

Drugs Used to Treat Thromboembolic Disorders

The QUESTION column and the ANSWER column have been offset so you can cover the answer while reading the question, allowing you to assess your knowledge.

Question	Answer
1. Differentiate among thromboembolic disease, thrombosis, thrombus, and embolus.	
2. Explain factors that trigger blood clot formation.	1. See textbook, p. 346.
3. List factor(s) that trigger(s) the intrinsic blood clotting pathway.	2. See textbook, p. 346.
4. Identify factor(s) that the extrinsic pathway triggers.	3. Factor XII
5. What is the difference between red and white blood clots?	4. Factor VII to VIIa (factor VIIa can also activate factor X)
6. Describe appropriate nonpharmacologic patient education for prevention and treatment of thromboembolic disease.	5. Red embolus is a venous thrombus. White thrombi develop in arteries. See also textbook, p. 347.
7. Differentiate among the drug actions of platelet inhibitors, anticoagulants, thrombolytic agents, and thromboembolic agents.	6. See textbook, p. 347.
8. Summarize the nursing actions that can help in the prevention of clot formation.	7. Thromboembolic agents either prevent platelet aggregation or inhibit a variety of steps in fibrin clot formation. Anticoagulants prevent new clot formation. Platelet inhibitors reduce arterial clot formation by inhibiting platelet aggregation. Thrombolytic agents dissolve thromboemboli already formed.
9. State nutritional information that should be provided to an individual for whom an anticoagulant is prescribed.	8. See textbook, p. 348.
10. Identify laboratory tests used to evaluate anticoagulant therapy.	9. See textbook, p. 348.
11. Explain the desired therapeutic outcomes for platelet inhibitors.	10. Textbook, anticoagulant monographs Prothrombin time (PT) is reported as International Normalized Ratio (INR) and is routinely used for warfarin therapy; APTT is most commonly used for heparin therapy.
12. List premedication assessments that should be performed before administering aspirin as a platelet inhibitor.	11. Reduce the frequency of TIAs, strokes, and myocardial infarction.

Copyright © 2001 by Mosby, Inc. All rights reserved.

13. What specific medication may be prescribed after cardiac valve replacement to prevent clot formation?

14. Differentiate the between the actions of low molecular weight heparins (LMWHs) and heparin.
15. What drug is used as an antidote in case of heparin overdose?

16. What laboratory studies are used to monitor for adverse effects of LMWHs?
17. What is the normal therapeutic range for warfarin therapy?

18. What is the antidote for hemorrhage that occurs with warfarin therapy?

12. Neurological assessment, gastrointestinal symptoms present, check for any concurrent anticoagulant therapy being taken; if on oral hypoglycemics, baseline serum glucose levels.
13. Dipyridamole (Persantine)

14. Heparin acts at several specific points in the coagulation pathway. LMWHs act at fewer specific steps in the coagulation pathway (factors Xa and thrombin), reducing the potential for hemorrhage. LMWHs also have a longer duration of action. Ardeparin, dalteparin, and enoxaparin have no antiplatelet activity and only minimal effect on PT and APTT.
15. Protamine sulfate; see textbook, p. 356 for details.

16. Periodic CBC, daily platelet counts, and periodic checking of stools for occult blood are tests used to monitor for adverse effects of LMWHs.
17. Prothrombin time (PT) is used to monitor warfarin therapy. PT is expressed as the INR. The optimal dosage of warfarin is that which prolongs the PT and maintains the INR at 2 to 3. In some medical conditions the INR may be maintained at 2.5 to 3.5.
18. In most cases of hemorrhage, the dosage of warfarin is withheld until the INR returns to therapeutic levels. In rare cases, Vitamin K is administered. In cases of severe hemorrhage, a transfusion with plasma or whole blood may be required.

Copyright © 2001 by Mosby, Inc. All rights reserved.

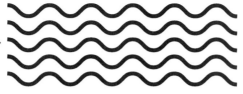

Practice Quiz

Drugs Used to Treat Thromboembolic Disorders

COMPLETION

Complete the following statements.

A(n) 1._____ is a circulating blood clot that may be trapped in a distal capillary causing an obstruction. A 2._____ is a stationary blood clot.

A class of drugs used to prevent blood clot formation is 3._____. The class of drugs used to dissolve recently formed thrombi is known as 4._____.

The therapeutic effect of heparin is monitored by the use of the laboratory test known as 5._____ time. The normal therapeutic range desired is 6._____. LMWHs (low molecular weight heparins) are monitored for adverse effect using the following laboratory tests: 7._____, 8._____, and 9._____.

Side effects to be reported when heparin therapy is used include: 10._____, 11._____, 12._____, and 13._____.

The antidote for excessive bleeding during warfarin therapy is 14._____.

MATCHING

Select the laboratory test(s) used to monitor the drug therapy listed.

_____ 15. Warfarin
_____ 16. Therapeutic effect of heparin
     a. Whole blood clotting time
     b. PT or INR
     c. APTT

CALCULATION

17. Ordered: 1000 ml D_5W with 10,000 U heparin added. Infuse at a rate of 80 U/hr IV. Set the infusion pump, calibrated in ml/hr, at _____ ml/hr.

18. Ordered: 1 liter $D_5W/0.9\%$ NaCl to infuse at 80 ml/hr. Using a microdrip administration set, at how many drops/minute should the infusion be set? _____

END-OF-CHAPTER MATH REVIEW

1. Ordered: Heparin 2000 U sc stat.
   On hand: Heparin 10,000 U /ml is available.
   Give: _____ ml.
2. Ordered: 100 ml 5% D/W with 30,000 U heparin.
   Infuse at a rate of 800 U/hr, IV. Set the infusion pump, calibrated in ml/hr, at _____ ml/hr.
   Three hours after the infusion is started, the physician changes the order to 1200 U/hr. How much heparin has already infused? _____ units.
   What rate would the infusion pump be adjusted to?
   Set infusion pump at: _____ ml/ hr.
3. Ordered: Persantine 75 mg per day qid.
   How many 75 mg tablets should the patient be dismissed with in order to take the medication for the next 7 days?
   Give: _____ tablets

CRITICAL THINKING QUESTIONS

1. A patient comes from surgery following a femoral bypass with a heparin drip running through a pump. What nursing assessments should be made to monitor this patient's postoperative progress? The operative record indicates she received a total of 50,000 U of heparin during the operative procedure. The postoperative orders do not state a specific rate of flow for the heparin drip that is currently running through the pump at 8 ml/hr. What actions should be taken by the nurse?
2. Review the procedure for administration of enoxaparin subcutaneously. What patient monitoring should be done during therapy with this drug?

Copyright © 2001 by Mosby, Inc.   All rights reserved.

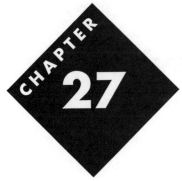

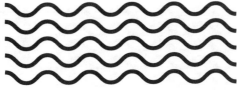

CHAPTER 27

Syllabus

Drugs Used to Treat Upper Respiratory Disease

CHAPTER CONTENTS

Upper Respiratory Tract Anatomy and Physiology
(p. 359)
Common Upper Respiratory Diseases (p. 360)
Treatment of Upper Respiratory Diseases (p. 362)
Drug Therapy for Upper Respiratory Diseases (p. 362)
Drug Class: Sympathomimetic Decongestants
(p. 363)
Drug Class: Antihistamines (p. 364)
Drug Class: Respiratory Anti-inflammatory Agents
(p. 366)

CHAPTER OBJECTIVES

1. State the causes of allergic rhinitis and nasal
    congestion.
2. Explain the major actions (effects) of
    sympathomimetic, antihistaminic, and corticosteroid
    decongestants and Cromolyn.
3. Define *rhinitis medicamentosa* and describe the
    patient education needed to prevent it.
4. Review the procedure for administration of
    medications by nose drops, sprays, and inhalation.
5. Explain why all decongestant products should be
    used cautiously in persons with hypertension,
    hyperthyroidism, diabetes mellitus, cardiac disease,
    increased intraocular pressure, or prostatic disease.
6. State the nursing assessments needed to monitor
    therapeutic response and development of side effects
    to expect or report from the use of decongestant drug
    therapy.
7. Identify essential components involved in planning
    patient education that will enhance compliance with
    the treatment regimen.

KEY WORDS

rhinitis
sinusitis
allergic rhinitis
antigen-antibody
histamine

rhinorrhea
decongestants
rhinitis medicamentosa
antihistamines
anti-inflammatory agents

ASSIGNMENTS

Read textbook pp. 359-367.
Study Key Words associated with chapter content.
Study Review Sheet for Chapter 27.
Complete End-of-Chapter Math Review and Critical
    Thinking Questions.
Complete Collaborative Activity as assigned by instructor.
Complete Chapter 27 Practice Quiz.
Complete Chapter 27 Exam.

COLLABORATIVE ACTIVITY

*Complete the following as preparation for in-class
discussion and group work that may be assigned by the
instructor.*

W.G., age 58, comes to the physician's office with
complaints of a large amount of cloudy nasal discharge, a
cough, headache, and "aching all over" the body. He has a
fever of 99.8° F.

The doctor prescribes phenylephrine (Neo-
Synephrine) nasal spray 0.25%, two sprays in each nostril
q 3-4 hours; ASA gr. 650 mg q 4 h for temperature above
100° F and relief of discomfort

What health education would you perform prior to
W.G.'s leaving the doctor's office?

Copyright © 2001 by Mosby, Inc.   All rights reserved.

CHAPTER 27

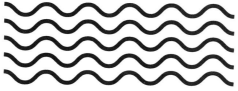

Review Sheet

Drugs Used to Treat Upper Respiratory Disease

and the ANSWER column have been offset so you can cover the answer while reading the question, allowing you to assess your knowledge.

Question

1. What is allergic rhinitis?
2. What are the drugs of choice for treating allergic rhinitis?
3. What is the mechanism of action of decongestants?
4. What is a "rebound" effect associated with nasally administered decongestants?

5. Name two commonly used decongestants administered intranasally, and two administered orally.

6. Explain how to administer a nasal spray, nose drops, and medications by inhalation.

7. What response does histamine release have on the mucous membranes?
8. What is an antigen?
9. When is histamine released?

10. How do antihistamines act?

11. What side effects can be anticipated whenever an antihistamine is administered?

12. What actions should be initiated to offset the drying effects of antihistamines?
13. What patient education should accompany the use of antihistamines?

Answer

1. Inflamed nasal mucosa associated with an allergic reaction.
2. Antihistamines
3. Decongestants are alpha adrenergic receptor stimulants that constrict blood vessels in the nasal passages, reducing swollen tissues and obstruction.
4. Excessive or prolonged use of nasal decongestants causes a rebound swelling in the nasal passages that requires further use of nasal decongestants to unblock nasal passages. It is difficult to break this cycle, so it is particularly important not to overuse nasal decongestants.
5. Pseudoephedrine (Sudafed)—oral tablets
    Phenylpropanolamine (Rhindecon)—oral tablets
    Phenylephrine (NeoSynephrine)—nasal spray
    Oxymetazoline (Afrin)—nasal spray
    Xylometazoline (Otrivin)—nasal spray
    See Table 27-1, p. 363.
6. See Chapter 10: Preparation and Administration of Medications by Percutaneous Routes, pp. 150-153.
7. Urticaria (itching), redness, and edema.
8. A substance that elicits an immunologic response such as the production of a specific antibody against that substance.
9. In cases of tissue damage (trauma), allergic reactions, and infection.
10. Histamines block the H_1 receptor sites on the target cells; they do not affect the amount or the release of histamine.
11. Sedation and dryness of mucous membranes (anticholinergic effects).
12. Consume an adequate fluid intake of 8–12 8 oz. glasses daily.

Copyright © 2001 by Mosby, Inc.   All rights reserved.

14. What is the action of cromolyn sodium (Nasalcrom)?

15. What condition is treated with cromolyn sodium (Nasalcrom) that affects the upper respiratory tract?

16. What are the desired therapeutic outcomes from the use of respiratory anti-inflammatory agents?

17. When a drug monograph says that a drug produces anticholinergic effects, what does this mean?

13. Maintain adequate hydration. If the person knows he/she is going to be exposed to an allergen (e.g., pollen outdoors), take the dose 30 to 45 minutes prior to possible exposure to block receptors before histamine can attach. If exposure is unanticipated, take a dose immediately upon recognition of an allergic response (e.g., runny nose and burning, itchy eyes). Exercise caution when operating any power equipment or while driving because of the medicine's sedative effects.

14. Cromolyn prevents release of histamine from its storage sites, the mast cells.

15. Cromolyn is used with other medications to treat severe allergic rhinitis and to prevent release of histamine that causes the symptoms of allergic rhinitis.

16. Reduction in rhinorrhea, rhinitis, itching, and sneezing.

17. Blurred vision; constipation; urinary retention; dryness of mucosa of mouth, throat, and nose.

Copyright © 2001 by Mosby, Inc. All rights reserved.

CHAPTER 27

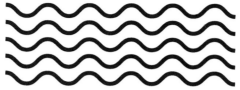

Practice Quiz

Drugs Used to Treat Upper Respiratory Disease

COMPLETION

Complete the following statements.

1. Decongestants cause the blood vessels in the nasal mucosa to _____.
2. Rhinitis medicamentosa can be prevented by _____.
3. The drug class of choice to treat the symptoms of allergic rhinitis is _____.
4. Cromolyn sodium should be administered _____.
5. The desired therapeutic outcomes from the use of respiratory anti-inflammatory agents (intranasal corticosteroids) is _____.

ESSAY

6. Explain the correct technique for administering nose drops and nasal spray.

CRITICAL THINKING QUESTIONS

1. J.L. has been using phenylephrine nasal drops 2-3 times per day for the past three weeks. He comes to the physician's office complaining that his symptoms are worse than when he initiated treatment. What assessments should the nurse make?
2. A.C. has been using chlorpheniramine maleate tablets three times per day and is now having considerable sedation. Her once productive cough has become nonproductive. What nursing actions should be considered?
3. A patient calls the office and asks the nurse how she can tell if her inhaler is almost empty. What would your response be?
4. Explain how to properly administer a medication by inhalation such as fluticasone, 2 sprays in each nostril once daily.
5. Perform health teaching for the proper administration of nose drops.

Copyright © 2001 by Mosby, Inc. All rights reserved.

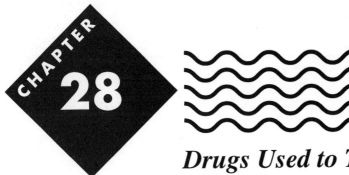

CHAPTER 28

Syllabus

Drugs Used to Treat Lower Respiratory Disease

CHAPTER CONTENTS

CHAPTER OBJECTIVES

1. Compare the physiologic responses of the respiratory system to emphysema, chronic bronchitis, and asthma.
2. Describe the physiology of respiration.
3. Identify the components of blood gases.
4. Cite nursing assessments used to evaluate the respiratory status of a patient.
5. Implement patient education for patients receiving drug therapy for lower respiratory disease.
6. Distinguish the mechanisms of action of expectorants, antitussives, and mucolytic agents.
7. Review the procedures for administration of medication by inhalation.
8. State the nursing assessments needed to monitor therapeutic response and the development of side effects to expect or report from expectorant, antitussive, and mucolytic therapy.
9. State the nursing assessments needed to monitor therapeutic response and development of side effects to expect or report from sympathomimetic bronchodilator therapy.

10. State the nursing assessments needed to monitor therapeutic response and development of side effects to expect or report from anticholinergic bronchodilator therapy.
11. List side effects known to occur with the use of xanthine derivatives, and correlate these with the needed nursing assessments and interventions.
12. State the nursing assessments needed to monitor therapeutic response and development of side effects to expect or report from corticosteroid inhalant therapy.

KEY WORDS

ventilation	oxygen saturation
perfusion	spirometry
diffusion	cough
goblet cells	asthma
obstructive airway disease	bronchitis
bronchospasm	emphysema
chronic obstructive	expectorants
pulmonary disease	antitussives
(COPD)	mucolytic agents
restrictive airway disease	bronchodilators
arterial blood gases	anti-inflammatory agents

ASSIGNMENTS

Read textbook pp. 368-396.
Study Key Words associated with chapter content.
Study Review Sheet for Chapter 28.
Complete End-of-Chapter Math Review and Critical
    Thinking Questions.
Complete Collaborative Activity as assigned by instructor.
Complete Chapter 28 Practice Quiz.
Complete Chapter 28 Exam.

Copyright © 2001 by Mosby, Inc.   All rights reserved.

COLLABORATIVE ACTIVITY

Complete the following as preparation for in-class discussion and group work that may be assigned by the instructor.

Research the effects of smoking on the respiratory tract. Include current statistics on the incidence of smoking in young people. Discuss cigarettes as addictive drugs and as entry drugs leading to marijuana and cocaine use.

Copyright © 2001 by Mosby, Inc.   All rights reserved.

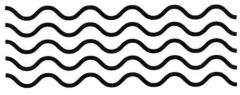

Review Sheet

Drugs Used to Treat Lower Respiratory Disease

The QUESTION column and the ANSWER column have been offset so that you can cover the answers while reading the questions, allowing you to assess your knowledge.

Question

1. What are the differences between obstructive and restrictive respiratory diseases?
2. Why are pulmonary function tests performed?

3. Why is the SAO_2 ratio valuable in an assessment of respiratory function?

4. What is asthma?

5. What is emphysema?

6. What is the action of expectorants?

7. What is the action of an antitussive agent?

8. What is the action of a mucolytic agent?
9. What is the purpose of administering a bronchodilator?

10. What types of drugs are known as anti-inflammatory agents?

11. What data should be collected as part of a respiratory assessment?

12. What dietary considerations should be made for a person with a respiratory disease?
13. How should persons with known respiratory disease prevent infection?

Answer

1. Obstructive disease is associated with narrowed air passages and increasing resistance to air flow (e.g., asthma, acute bronchitis). Restrictive airway disease is characterized by restricted alveolar expansion due to loss of elasticity of tissue or physical deformity of the chest itself.
2. To assess ventilation and diffusion capacity of the lungs and to determine whether medicines are having a therapeutic effect.
3. It reflects the percent of oxygen bound to the hemoglobin compared with the maximum amount of oxygen that could be attached.
4. Asthma is a chronic inflammatory disease of bronchi and bronchioles.
5. Emphysema is a disease of alveolar destruction without fibrosis.
6. Expectorants liquefy mucus by stimulating natural lubricant fluids.
7. Antitussives suppress the cough center in the brain.
8. Mucolytic agents reduce stickiness and viscosity of pulmonary secretions by acting directly on mucus plug to cause dissolution.
9. It causes a widening of the opening of the bronchioles and alveolar ducts and a decrease in resistance to airflow into the alveolar sacs.
10. Corticosteroids are the most effective anti-inflammatory agents. Other agents are leukotriene modifiers, cromolyn, and nedocromil.
11. See textbook, pp. 373, 376.

12. Well-balanced diet to maintain near-normal weight. With dyspnea eat small servings throughout day, take small bites, and eat slowly. Administer oxygen during meals as needed.

Copyright © 2001 by Mosby, Inc.   All rights reserved.

14. What medication administration considerations should be made for the delivery of aerosol therapy to a child or elderly person?
15. Review the premedication assessments associated with acetylcysteine therapy.
16. What types of patients benefit from bronchodilator therapy?
17. What two classes of drugs are prescribed as bronchodilators?
18. How do sympathomimetic (adrenergic) agents act?
19. Which drugs are classified as xanthine derivatives?

20. How do xanthines work?

21. What pharmacologic effects do xanthines cause?

22. How can dosages of theophylline be measured?

23. Cite important aspects of patient education and health promotion for individuals with a lower respiratory disease.
24. What posture does a dyspneic patient assume?
25. Describe appropriate health teaching for patients requiring respiratory therapy.

26. What precautions must be used when administering an iodine product?
27. When should SSKI not be administered?

28. What types of respiratory diseases may be treated with mucolytic agents [e.g., acetylcysteine (Mucomyst)]?

29. The patient receiving medication by inhalation should be placed in what position?
30. The patient should be instructed to exhale through _____ lips.
31. What patient teaching should be performed for a patient taking an expectorant?
32. What is the desired action for giving saline solution by nebulizer?

33. What classes of antitussive agents are available?

13. Good hygiene; influenza and pneumococcal vaccinations. Seek medical attention at earliest signs of suspected infection.
14. See textbook, p. 337.

15. See textbook, p. 381.

16. Patients with diseases that cause constriction of the tracheobronchial tree, obstructing the airways.
17. Sympathomimetics and xanthine derivatives.
18. Adrenergic agents stimulate beta$_2$ receptors, causing bronchodilation. Many of the drugs also stimulate beta$_1$ receptors in the heart. Always monitor patients taking adrenergic agents for changes in cardiac function (e.g., hypertension, tachycardia), CNS stimulation (exhibited as insomnia, nervousness, anxiety, tremors), and gastrointestinal (GI) disturbances.
19. Aminophylline, theophylline, dyphylline, oxtriphylline. (Note: all xanthine derivatives except caffeine end in "-phylline".)
20. They cause an increase in cyclic adenosine monophosphate (AMP), a substance that is associated with bronchodilation and smooth muscle relaxation.
21. They stimulate the CNS, cause diuresis, increase gastric secretions, and stimulate the heart to beat rapidly. Always monitor patients for nausea, changes in cardiac function, and CNS stimulation.
22. Theophylline levels can be monitored by a blood test. Adult: 10-20 mcg/ml; Newborn: 6-11 mcg/ml.

23. See textbook, pp. 377-378.
24. Sits upright and leans forward from the waist, resting the elbows on the knees. When hospitalized, will be placed in a high Fowler's position.
25. See pp. 377-378, Patient Education and Health Promotion.
26. Dilute in water or fruit juice. Use a straw placed well back on the tongue to administer iodine products; this prevents permanent staining of the teeth.
27. Do *not* give to a patient allergic to iodine or to one who has hyperthyroidism, hyperkalemia, or experiences a skin eruption after taking the medication.
28. Emphysema, bronchitis, pneumonia

29. Sitting

30. Pursed

31. Teach the patient the difference between a productive and nonproductive cough, as well as measures to combat nonproductive coughs.
32. Hydration of viscous mucus

Copyright © 2001 by Mosby, Inc. All rights reserved.

34. What are the major drawbacks to using an opiate antitussive?
35. In what type of patient must great caution be exercised if an opiate antitussive is to be administered?
36. Give one example of an antitussive agent.

37. What premedication assessments should be made prior to administering an antitussive agent, mucolytic agent, expectorant, anticholinergic bronchodilating agent, xanthine derivative bronchodilating agent, respiratory anti-inflammatory agent, and antileukotriene agents?
38. What are the four components of asthma therapy?

33. Opiate and nonopiate cough suppressants.

34. Codeine may cause dependence (rarely), respiratory depression, bronchial constriction, central nervous system (CNS) depression, and constipation.

35. Patients with preexisting pulmonary distress; persons already taking sedative/hypnotics, CNS depressants, or psychotropic agents; persons using alcohol.

36. Codeine

37. Antitussive agent, pp. 380-381.
Mucolytic agents, p. 381.
Anticholinergic bronchodilating agents, p. 384.
Xanthine derivative bronchodilating agents, p. 385.
Respiratory anti-inflammatory agents, p. 386.
Antileukotriene agents, p. 389.

38. Patient education, environmental control, comprehensive pharmacologic therapy, and objective monitoring via regular use of a peak flow meter.

Drugs Used to Treat Lower Respiratory Disease

DEFINITIONS

Define the following terms.
1. Perfusion:

2. Ventilation:

3. Bronchitis:

4. Emphysema:

5. Expectorants (action):

6. Antitussives (action):

7. Mucolytics (action):

ESSAY

8. When the clinical instructor sends you to do a respiratory assessment, what nursing actions would you perform?
9. What effect does smoking have on theophylline therapy?
10. What premedication assessments should be performed before administering an xanthine derivative bronchodilating agent?
11. What drugs are used in the treatment of asthma on a short-term and long-term basis?
12. What are the pharmacologic effects of the antileukotrienes?

END-OF-CHAPTER MATH REVIEW

1. Ordered: Diphenhydramine (Benylin) 25 mg q 4 h
   On hand: Diphenhydramine (Benylin) 13.3 mg/5 ml
   Give: _____ ml or _____ tsp.
2. Ordered: Terbutaline (Brethine) 0.25 mg sc
   On hand: Terbutaline 1 mg/ml
   Give: _____ml.
3. Ordered: Theophylline Elixir 9 mg/kg/24 hrs in 4 divided doses
   The patient weighs 86 lbs.
   Give: _____ mg per individual dose
4. On hand: Theophylline Elixir 50 mg/5 ml
   Give: _____ml per individual dose

CRITICAL THINKING QUESTIONS

1. Explain why the action of a beta adrenergic blocking agent may interfere with the therapeutic effects of bronchodilating agents [e.g., albuterol (Proventil)].
2. Differentiate among the actions of acetylcysteine, guaifenesin, and potassium iodide on mucus in the respiratory tract.

Copyright © 2001 by Mosby, Inc.   All rights reserved.

CHAPTER 29

Syllabus

Drugs Used to Treat Oral Disorders

CHAPTER CONTENT

Mouth Disorders (p. 391)
Drug Therapy of Mouth Disorders (p. 393)
    Drug Class: Dentifrices (p. 395)
    Drug Class: Mouthwashes (p. 396)

CHAPTER OBJECTIVES

1. Cite the treatment alternatives and associated nursing assessments to monitor response to drug therapy for common mouth disorders.
2. Identify baseline data the nurse should collect on a continuous basis for comparison and evaluation of drug effectiveness.
3. Identify important nursing assessments and interventions associated with the drug therapy and treatment of diseases of the mouth.

KEY WORDS

cold sores	tartar
fever blisters	gingivitis
canker sores	halitosis
candidiasis	xerostomia
stomatitis	dentifrice
plaque	mouthwashes
dental caries	

ASSIGNMENTS

Read textbook pp. 391-396.
Study Key Words associated with chapter content.
Study Review Sheet for Chapter 29.
Complete End-of-Chapter Critical Thinking Question.
Complete Chapter 29 Practice Quiz.
Complete Chapter 29 Exam.

Copyright © 2001 by Mosby, Inc.   All rights reserved.

Review Sheet

Drugs Used to Treat Oral Disorders

The QUESTION column and the ANSWER column have been offset so that you can cover the answers while reading the questions, allowing you to assess your knowledge.

Question	Answer
1. Cite the major goals of treatment and drug therapy used for cold sores, canker sores, stomatitis, plaque, halitosis, and xerostomia.	
2. Explain how to perform an assessment of the oral cavity.	1. See textbook, p. 393.
3. Cite basic nursing interventions used for cold sores, canker sores, stomatitis, plaque, halitosis, xerostomia, and denture wearers.	2. See textbook, p. 394.
4. What types of mouthwashes should be recommended for use to: a. reduce plaque accumulation and gingivitis? b. treat oral stomatitis? c. decrease bleeding or irritation?	3. See textbook, pp. 394-395.
5. When lidocaine, a local anesthetic, is used as an oral spray or as a viscous solution, what precautions should be taught to the patient?	4. a. Medicinal mouthwashes (e.g., Listerine) b. Chlorhexidine (Peridex) c. Mouthwashes containing zinc chloride
6. Describe the stomatitis scale.	5. Do not smoke, eat, or drink for at least 30 minutes after use. Test ability to swallow before taking oral foods or drink. These products decrease normal sensations in the mouth, test temperature of foods or drinks before ingesting to prevent accidental burning of the oral mucosa.
	6. See textbook, p. 392.

Copyright © 2001 by Mosby, Inc.   All rights reserved.

Practice Quiz

Drugs Used to Treat Oral Disorders

DEFINITIONS

Define the following terms.

1. Fever blisters:

2. Candidiasis:

3. Halitosis:

4. Xerostomia:

List five medicines that may be used to treat stomatitis.

5. _____

6. _____

7. _____

8. _____

9. _____

CRITICAL THINKING QUESTION

1. Compare oral hygiene measures appropriate in a person with a healthy mouth verses those measures needed in a person with a moderate to severe mouth disorder.

Copyright © 2001 by Mosby, Inc.   All rights reserved.

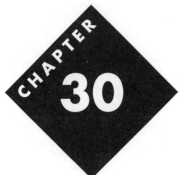

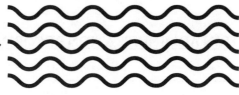

Syllabus

Drugs Used to Treat Gastroesophageal Reflux and Peptic Ulcer Disease

CHAPTER CONTENT

CHAPTER OBJECTIVES

1. Cite common stomach disorders that require drug therapy.
2. Identify factors that prevent breakdown of the body's normal defense barriers resulting in ulcer formation.
3. State the drug classifications and actions used to treat stomach disorders.
4. Develop health teaching for an individual with stomach disorders that incorporates pharmacologic and nonpharmacologic treatment modalities.

KEY WORDS

parietal cells
hydrochloric acid
gastroesophageal reflux
    disease (GERD)
heartburn
peptic ulcer disease (PUD)
Helicobacter pylori

ASSIGNMENTS

Read textbook pp. 396-410.
Study Key Words associated with chapter content.
Study Review Sheet for Chapter 30.
Complete End-of-Chapter Math Review and Critical
    Thinking Questions.
Complete Collaborative Activities as assigned by
    instructor.
Complete Chapter 30 Practice Quiz.
Complete Chapter 30 Exam.

COLLABORATIVE ACTIVITIES

Complete the following as preparation for in-class discussion and group work that may be assigned by the instructor.

F.W. develops diarrhea after taking a prescribed antacid for five days.

1. What type of antacids may initiate diarrhea?
2. What nursing diagnosis should be initiated on F.W.'s care plan?
3. F.W. is also taking digoxin 0.25 mg daily and levodopa 1 gm qid.
   Using the MAR record on the next page or one distributed by the instructor, develop a time schedule for the administration of the drugs ordered.
4. When levodopa, digoxin, and an antacid are prescribed together, what nursing assessments should be performed?

Copyright © 2001 by Mosby, Inc.   All rights reserved.

MARTINDALE HOMETOWN HOSPITAL

MEDICATION ADMINISTRATION RECORD

NAME: RM-BD: Init   Signature   Title
 ID NO.:   AGE:
 DIAGNOSIS: SEX:

PHYSICIAN: Ht: Wt:

SCHEDULED MEDICATIONS

DATE	MEDICATION-STRENGTH-FORM-ROUTE	0030-0729	0730-1529	1530-0029

** PRN MEDICATIONS**

Copyright © 2001 by Mosby, Inc.   All rights reserved.

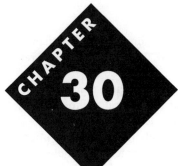

30

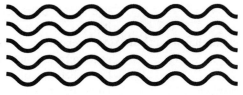

Review Sheet

Drugs Used to Treat Gastroesophageal Reflux and Peptic Ulcer Disease

The QUESTION column and the ANSWER column have been offset so that you can cover the answers while reading the questions, allowing you to assess your knowledge.

Question	**Answer**
1. What types of conditions are treated with antacids?	
2. What is the difference between gastroesophageal reflux disease (GERD) and peptic ulcer disease?	1. Antacids decrease hyperacidity associated with PUD, GERD, gastritis, and hiatal hernia.
3. What are the major treatment goals for GERD and peptic ulcer disease?	2. See textbook, pp. 397-398.
4. What premedication assessments should be made prior to beginning antacid therapy?	3. See textbook, p. 398.
5. What effect does the administration of an antacid have on the pH of the gastric secretions?	4. Prior to antacid therapy check for any abnormal renal function. If present avoid magnesium-containing products. Check bowel pattern for diarrhea or constipation. Record any gastric pain or symptoms present. If patient is pregnant or has edema, heart failure, hypertension, or salt restrictions, ensure that a low-sodium antacid is prescribed. Check scheduling of antacids in relation to other prescribed medications to avoid interactions.
6. Are antacids alkaline or acidic?	5. Antacids buffer the hydrogen ion concentration, reducing the acidity of the gastric secretions and raising the pH of the gastric contents to neutralize gastric secretions.
7. Describe effect(s) of the following active ingredients of antacids: simethicone aluminum hydroxide magnesium oxide or hydroxide magnesium trisilicate calcium carbonate	6. Mildly alkaline
8. What ingredients in an antacid may produce constipation?	7. Simethicone is an antiflatulent. Aluminum hydroxide, magnesium oxide and hydroxide, magnesium trisilicate, and calcium carbonate all buffer gastric acidity.
9. What ingredients in antacids may cause diarrhea?	8. Calcium and aluminum products may cause constipation.
10. What ingredient(s) in antacids should not be administered to patients with renal disease?	9. Magnesium

Copyright © 2001 by Mosby, Inc.   All rights reserved.

11. Define *acid rebound.*

12. Should antacids be given on an empty stomach or with food in the stomach?

13. What types of products can produce a systemic alkaline effect?

14. Patients with chronic renal failure who have hyperphosphatemia can benefit from taking which type of antacid and why?

15. What class of antibiotics, when given with antacids (Mg, Ca, or Al types), interact to result in a decrease in the absorption of the antibiotic?

16. Because antacids alter the absorption rate of digoxin, digitoxin, and iron compounds, what dosing schedule should be used to administer antacids when these medicines are also ordered?

17. In order to obtain the most rapid onset of action, should an antacid be administered in a liquid or a tablet form?

18. Are antacid tablets recommended for the treatment of peptic ulcer disease?

19. Compare the actions of antihistamines and H_2 antagonists.

20. What premedication assessments should be performed for H_2 antagonists?

21. When should the H_2 antagonist agents, cimetidine (Tagamet), famotidine (Pepcid), nizatidine (Axid), or ranitidine (Zantac) be administered in relation to food intake?

22. Compare the dosage and scheduling of the H_2 antagonists.

23. If antacid therapy is continued concurrently with the use of cimetidine (Tagamet), what scheduling for the antacid should be used?

24. What advantages does famotidine (Pepcid) have when compared to cimetidine (Tagamet)?

10. Magnesium should not be administered to patients with renal failure because they are unable to excrete it.

11. Acid rebound is found with calcium compounds and sodium bicarbonate; acid is neutralized followed by hypersecretion of gastric acid.

12. Given on an empty stomach, the neutralizing effects of antacids last only approximately 30 minutes. With food in the stomach, the neutralizing action is extended to 2 to 4 hours.

13. Sodium bicarbonate (baking soda)

14. Aluminum hydroxide and aluminum carbonate gel, because the aluminum ion binds the phosphate in the gastrointestinal tract.

15. Tetracyclines

16. Administer 1 hour before or 2 hours after the antacid.

17. Liquid form

18. Tablets do not contain enough antacid to be effective for treatment of peptic ulcers.

19. Antihistamines block the receptor sites on target cells (e.g., arterioles, capillaries, glands) so that the histamine cannot attach there. This prevents the symptoms of an allergic reaction such as rhinorrhea and lacrimation. To be effective, antihistamines need to be taken 30-40 minutes before exposure to allergens such as pollen or as soon as symptoms first appear. Antihistamines do not have a direct effect on gastric acid secretion. H_2 antagonists (e.g., cimetidine, famotidine, nizatidine, ranitidine) block the action of histamine on the gastric acid-secreting cells (parietal cells) in the stomach.

20. See textbook p. 402. Assess patient's mental status to detect CNS alterations, particularly with cimetidine therapy.

21. Cimetidine, famotidine, and ranitidine are administered with food. Nizatidine may be administered with or without food.

22. Cimetidine (Tagamet) 300 mg, 4 times per day with meals and at bedtime; famotidine (Pepcid) 40 mg once daily at bedtime or 20 mg twice daily; ranitidine (Zantac) 150 mg, twice daily or 300 mg at bedtime. Nizatidine (Axid) po 300 mg, once daily at bedtime or 150 mg two times daily.

23. Antacids should be administered 1 hour before or 2 hours after the H_2 antagonist.

Copyright © 2001 by Mosby, Inc. All rights reserved.

25. How does the coating agent sucralfate (Carafate), differ from histamine H$_2$ antagonists?

26. List the actions of gastrointestinal prostaglandins.

27. What premedication assessments should be performed before misoprostol therapy?

28. Cite the most common side effect of misoprostol therapy.

29. How can diarrhea associated with misoprostol therapy be minimized?
30. Should misoprostol be taken during pregnancy?

31. What drugs can have altered absorption as a result of a reduction in gastric acid secretions?
32. What is the action of metoclopramide (Reglan)?

24. Famotidine is taken once daily, does not produce gynecomastia, and has fewer significant drug interactions reported with its use.
25. Coating agents do not affect the amount of hydrochloric acid secreted; they adhere to the crater of the ulcer.
26. Gastrointestinal prostaglandins stimulate GI motility, gastric acid and pepsin secretion, and protect the stomach and duodenal lining against ulceration.
27. Determine if the patient is pregnant. This drug is a uterine stimulant and may induce a miscarriage. Check pattern of bowel elimination. Misoprostol may induce diarrhea.
28. Diarrhea

29. Take misoprostol with meals and at bedtime; avoid antacids containing magnesium (e.g., Maalox, Mylanta).
30. Discontinue if that patient is pregnant.

31. Digoxin, ketoconazole, ampicillin, and iron
32. Metoclopramide is a gastric stimulant thought to block dopamine in the chemoreceptor trigger zone. It increases stomach contractions, relaxes the pyloric valve, and increases peristalsis in GI tract resulting in increased rate of gastric emptying and intestinal transit.

Copyright © 2001 by Mosby, Inc. All rights reserved.

CHAPTER 30

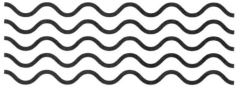

Practice Quiz

Drugs Used to Treat Gastroesophageal Reflux and Peptic Ulcer Disease

TRUE OR FALSE

Mark each statement "T" for true and "F" for false.
Correct all false statements.

_____ 1. Antacid tablets are effective in treating peptic ulcer disease.

_____ 2. Patients with renal failure may develop hypermagnesemia if magnesium-containing antacids are taken.

_____ 3. The pH of the stomach decreases when the hydrochloric acid content is reduced.

_____ 4. Smoking causes an increase in hydrochloric acid secretion.

_____ 5. Premedication assessments needed with misoprostol (Cytotec) include checking to see if the individual is pregnant and checking the normal pattern of bowel elimination.

_____ 6. The desired therapeutic outcome with omeprazole (Prilosec) is a reduction in heartburn and discomfort and healing of irritated gastrointestinal mucosa.

_____ 7. Sucralfate (Carafate) decreases gastric secretions.

_____ 8. Metoclopramide (Reglan) should be prescribed for nausea and vomiting associated with chemotherapy because it decreases peristalsis.

_____ 9. Antacids containing magnesium may be dangerous to patients with renal disease.

ESSAY

10. Name two antispasmodic agents.
11. Compare the daily dosages and side effects of cimetidine, ranitidine, and famotidine.

CALCULATIONS

12. Ordered: famotidine (Pepcid) 20 mg po bid
    On hand: famotidine (Pepcid) suspension 40 mg/5 ml
    Give: _____ ml.

13. Ordered: propantheline (Pro-Banthine) 15 mg ac and 30 mg at hs
    On hand: propantheline (Pro-Banthine) 15 mg tablets
    The ac dose will require _____ tablets and the hs dose will require _____ tablets.

END-OF-CHAPTER MATH REVIEW

1. Ordered: Ranitidine (Zantac) 50 mg in 100 ml D_5W IV over 20 minutes.
   Using an infusion pump, calibrated in ml/hr, at what rate would the infusion pump be set?
   _____ ml/hr

2. Ordered: Pepcid 35 mg po stat
   On hand: Pepcid 40 mg/ml oral suspension.
   Give _____ ml

CRITICAL THINKING QUESTIONS

1. Situation: J.C., age 45, has PUD and seems unaware that lifestyle changes are needed to treat the disorder. She has an H_2 antagonist ordered. What teaching approaches would be appropriate for her?

2. Situation: M.W. is complaining of intermittent diarrhea. No physical basis for the diarrhea has been identified. She also complains of heartburn. Explore self-treatments available with over-the-counter medicines that could cause the diarrhea.

Copyright © 2001 by Mosby, Inc.   All rights reserved.

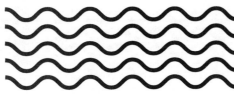

Syllabus

Drugs Used to Treat Nausea and Vomiting

CHAPTER CONTENT

Nausea and Vomiting (p. 410)
Common Causes of Nausea and Vomiting (p. 411)
Drug Therapy for Selected Causes of Nausea and
 Vomiting (p. 412)
 Drug Class: Dopamine Antagonists (p. 415)
 Drug Class: Serotonin Antagonists (p. 415)
 Drug Class: Anticholinergic Agents (p. 420)
 Drug Class: Corticosteroids (p. 420)
 Drug Class: Benzodiazepines (p. 421)
 Drug Class: Cannabinoids (p. 421)

CHAPTER OBJECTIVES

1. Compare the purposes of using antiemetic products.
2. State the therapeutic classes of antiemetics.
3. Discuss scheduling of antiemetics for maximum
   benefit.

KEY WORDS

postoperative nausea and
  vomiting (PONV)
chemotherapy-induced
  emesis (CIE)

hyperemesis gravidarum
anticipatory nausea and
  vomiting
delayed emesis

ASSIGNMENTS

Read textbook pp. 410-422.
Study Key Words associated with chapter content.
Study Review Sheet for Chapter 31.
Complete End-of-Chapter Math Review and Critical
  Thinking Questions.
Complete Collaborative Activities as assigned by
  instructor.
Complete Chapter 31 Practice Quiz.
Complete Chapter 31 Exam.

COLLABORATIVE ACTIVITIES

*Complete the following as preparation for in-class
discussion and group work that may be assigned by the
instructor.*
1. What is the usual dosage scheduling of serotonin
   antagonists in relation to a prescribed dose of
   chemotherapy?
2. What premedication assessments should be
   completed and recorded prior to administering a
   serotonin antagonist?

Copyright © 2001 by Mosby, Inc.   All rights reserved.

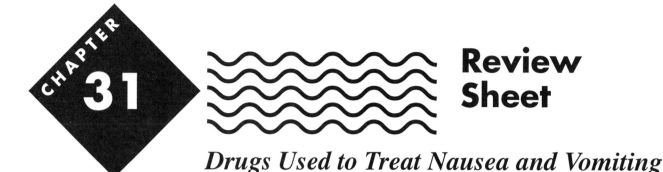

CHAPTER 31

Review Sheet

Drugs Used to Treat Nausea and Vomiting

The QUESTION column and the ANSWER column have been offset so that you can cover the answers while reading the questions, allowing you to assess your knowledge.

Question	**Answer**
1. What is an antiemetic?	
2. What six classes of drugs are used to treat nausea and vomiting?	1. A medication used to prevent nausea and vomiting
3. What is the mechanism of action for the six drug classes used to treat nausea and vomiting?	2. Dopamine antagonists, serotonin antagonists, anticholinergic agents, corticosteroids, benzodiazepines, and cannabinoids
	3. See sections labeled action for each drug class.
4. Name the most widely used antiemetic in the phenothiazine class used to treat nausea and vomiting associated with surgery, radiation, and cancer chemotherapy?	
5. What is the action of metoclopramide (Reglan) on the gastrointestinal tract that makes it useful as an antiemetic?	4. Prochlorperazine (Compazine)
6. When is ondansetron (Zofran) administered in relation to chemotherapy?	5. Metoclopramide is thought to work as an antiemetic by blocking dopamine in the chemoreceptor trigger zone. It has also been suggested that it inhibits serotonin when administered in higher doses.
7. What drugs are recommended for nausea and vomiting associated with pregnancy?	6. Ondansetron (Zofran) is administered 30 minutes before chemotherapy and at 4-hour intervals after chemotherapy for 2 doses.
8. What are the usual nursing implementations used for an adult and for an infant?	7. Administration of meclizine, cyclizine, or dimenhydrinate is recommended first for nausea and vomiting associated with pregnancy.
9. What are the usual premedication assessments performed for any antiemetic?	8. See textbook p. 414.
10. Define *hyperemesis gravidarum, psychogenic vomiting, anticipatory vomiting,* and *chemotherapy-induced vomiting.*	9. See textbook p. 413.
	10. See textbook p. 413.

Copyright © 2001 by Mosby, Inc. All rights reserved.

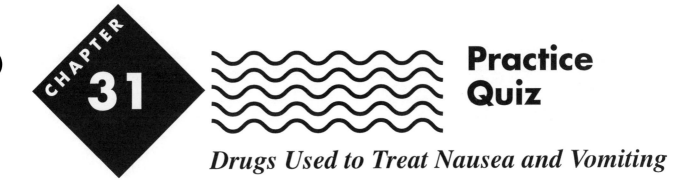

CHAPTER 31

Practice Quiz

Drugs Used to Treat Nausea and Vomiting

DEFINITIONS

Define the following terms.
1. Hyperemesis gravidarum:
2. Psychogenic vomiting:

COMPLETION

Complete the following statements.
3. CIE is an abbreviation for _____.

Antiemetics act by:
4. _____
5. _____
6. Dopamine antagonists act by:
   _____.
7. Ondansetron (Zofran) or granisetron (Kytril) are generally prescribed for _____ and _____-type vomiting.
8. Anticholinergic agents such as Dramamine are generally prescribed for _____-type vomiting.

ESSAY

9. When should an antiemetic be administered to a patient having postoperative nausea?
10. What is the cause of motion sickness?
11. How long after administration of chemotherapy can it take for delayed emesis to occur?
12. What six classes of drugs are used to treat nausea and vomiting?
13. What information should be included in a nursing assessment performed on a patient having nausea and vomiting?
14. Compare the premedication assessments listed for each of the six drug classes used in the treatment of nausea and vomiting.

END-OF-CHAPTER MATH REVIEW

1. Ordered: Ondansetron (Zofran) 0.15 mg/kg IV in 50 ml D_5W over 20 minutes before chemotherapy. The client's weight today is 135 lbs.
   Weight is: _____ kg
   The total amount of ondansetron to administer is _____?
   When administering this order using an infusion pump calibrated in ml/hr, set the pump at _____ml/hr.
2. Ordered: Dexamethasone 6 mg by IM injection stat. On hand: Dexamethasone 4mg/ml.
   Give: _____ ml

CRITICAL THINKING QUESTIONS

1. R.T., age 65, has been vomiting intermittently for 3 days with the "flu." He is a resident on your unit in the nursing home. What data should be collected and reported to the physician for further evaluation and action?
2. T.L. has been vomiting repeatedly following administration of chemotherapy and received metoclopramide an hour ago. What is the action of this drug and what further actions by the nurse are appropriate?

Copyright © 2001 by Mosby, Inc.   All rights reserved.   **159**

CHAPTER 32

Drugs Used to Treat Constipation and Diarrhea

Syllabus

CHAPTER CONTENT

Constipation (p. 423)
Diarrhea (p. 423)
    Drug Therapy for Constipation and Diarrhea (p. 425)
    Drug Class: Laxatives (p. 425)
    Drug Class: Antidiarrheal Agents (p. 426)

CHAPTER OBJECTIVES

1. State the underlying causes of constipation.
2. Explain the meaning of "normal" bowel habits.
3. Identify the indications for use, method of action, and onset of action for contact or stimulant laxatives, saline laxatives, lubricant or emollient laxatives, bulk-forming laxatives, and fecal softeners.
4. Describe medical conditions in which laxatives should not be used.
5. List nine causes of diarrhea.
6. State the differences between locally acting and systemically acting antidiarrheal agents.
7. Identify electrolytes that should be monitored whenever prolonged or severe diarrhea is present.
8. Describe nursing assessments needed to evaluate the state of hydration in patients suffering from either constipation or dehydration.
9. Cite conditions that generally respond favorably to antidiarrheal agents.
10. Prepare a list of medications that may cause diarrhea.

KEY WORDS

constipation
diarrhea
laxative

ASSIGNMENTS

Read textbook pp. 422-429.
Study Key Words associated with chapter content.
Study Review Sheet for Chapter 32.
Complete End-of-Chapter Critical Thinking Questions.
Complete Collaborative Activity as assigned by instructor.
Complete Chapter 32 Practice Quiz.
Complete Chapter 32 Exam.

COLLABORATIVE ACTIVITY

Complete the following as preparation for in-class discussion and group work that may be assigned by the instructor.

Explain the health teaching needed for an elderly patient who consistently takes one or more laxatives daily.

Copyright © 2001 by Mosby, Inc. All rights reserved.

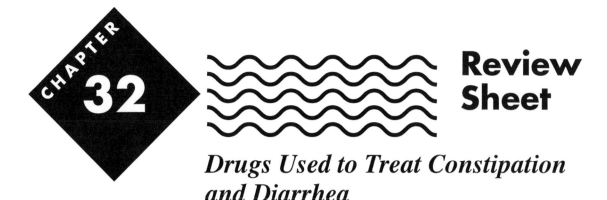

Drugs Used to Treat Constipation and Diarrhea

The QUESTION column and the ANSWER column have been offset so that you can cover the answers while reading the questions, allowing you to assess your knowledge.

Question

1. What is the mechanism of action of
   a. contact or stimulant laxatives?
   b. saline laxatives?
   c. lubricant or emollient laxatives?
   d. bulk-producing laxatives?
   e. fecal softeners?

2. What is the onset of action for
   a. contact or stimulant laxatives?
   b. saline laxatives?
   c. lubricant or emollient laxatives?
   d. bulk-producing laxatives?
   e. fecal softeners?

3. When administering fecal softeners, what factors must be considered to promote the action of these laxative agents?

4. Differentiate between the action of systemic and local antidiarrheal agents.

5. What premedication assessments should be performed before administration of an antidiarrheal agent?

6. Examine Table 32-1 to identify the names and types of laxatives commonly prescribed and Table 32-2 for antidiarrheals prescribed.

Answer

1. a. Promote peristalsis by irritation.
   b. Attract water into intestines from surrounding tissues, promote peristalsis.
   c. Lubricate intestinal wall and soften the stool, peristalsis does not appear to be increased.
   d. Cause water to be retained in stool, thus increasing bulk that stimulates peristalsis.
   e. Draw water into stool causing it to soften. No stimulation of peristalsis.

2. a. 6-10 hours orally; 60-90 minutes rectally
   b. 1-3 hours
   c. 6-8 hours
   d. 12-24 hours, up to 72 hours
   e. up to 72 hours

3. Adequate fluid intake is essential.

4. Systemic: Decrease peristalsis and GI mobility via the autonomic nervous system (ANS), allowing the mucosal lining to absorb nutrients, water, and electrolytes and leaving a formed stool from the residue remaining in the colon. Local: Adsorb excess water to cause a formed stool and to adsorb irritants or bacteria that cause diarrhea.

5. Take medication history and examine for drugs that may be contributing to the diarrhea; review for precipitating factors.

6. See textbook, pp. 427-428.

Copyright © 2001 by Mosby, Inc. All rights reserved.

Practice Quiz

Drugs Used to Treat Constipation and Diarrhea

COMPLETION

Complete the following statements.

Describe the mechanism of action of the following.

1. Bulk-producing laxatives:

2. Lubricant or emollient laxatives:

3. Locally acting antidiarrheal agents:

4. Systemic acting antidiarrheal agents:

5. What are the most common causes of intestinal infections?

6. What type of diet should be used to treat constipation?

7. What ingredient in antacid products is known to cause diarrhea?

8. What type of laxative is the drug of choice for treatment of persons requiring regular use of laxatives?

CRITICAL THINKING QUESTIONS

1. The physician asks a nurse to instruct the mother of a 6-month old infant on the procedure to insert a glycerin suppository. What information would you give?

2. An 80-year-old resident asks for a laxative daily. What health teaching should be done? Would you give the prn laxative daily?

Copyright © 2001 by Mosby, Inc.   All rights reserved.

Drugs Used to Treat Diabetes Mellitus

CHAPTER CONTENTS

CHAPTER OBJECTIVES

1. State the current definition of diabetes mellitus.
2. Identify the incidence of the disease in the United States.
3. Describe the current classification system for diabetes mellitus.
4. Differentiate between the symptoms of type 1 (formerly IDDM) and type 2 (formerly NIDDM) diabetes mellitus.
5. Identify the objectives of dietary control of diabetes mellitus.
6. Discuss the action and use of insulin as opposed to oral hypoglycemic and antihyperglycemic agents to control diabetes mellitus.
7. Identify the major nursing considerations associated with the management of diabetes (such as nutritional evaluation, dietary prescription, activity and exercise, and psychologic considerations).
8. Differentiate among the signs, symptoms, and management of hypoglycemia and hyperglycemia.
9. Discuss the contributing factors of, nursing assessments for, and nursing interventions for patients exhibiting complications associated with diabetes mellitus.

10. Develop a health teaching plan for persons taking any type of insulin or oral hypoglycemic agent.

KEY WORDS

diabetes mellitus
type 1 diabetes mellitus
type 2 diabetes mellitus
neuropathies
paresthesia
gestational diabetes
   mellitus

impaired glucose tolerance
   (IGT)
impaired fasting glucose
   (IFG)
hypoglycemia
hyperglycemia

ASSIGNMENTS

Read textbook pp. 430-449.
Study Key Words associated with chapter content.
Study Review Sheet for Chapter 33.
Complete End-of-Chapter Math Review and Critical
   Thinking Questions.
Complete Collaborative Activities as assigned by
   instructor.
Complete Chapter 33 Practice Quiz.
Complete Chapter 33 Exam.

COLLABORATIVE ACTIVITIES

Complete the following as preparation for in-class discussion and group work that may be assigned by the instructor.

1. Practice mixing short- and intermediate-acting insulin in the same syringe using the technique taught in your educational setting.
2. Explain the treatment(s) of hypoglycemia in response to excessive insulin intake.

Copyright © 2001 by Mosby, Inc.   All rights reserved.

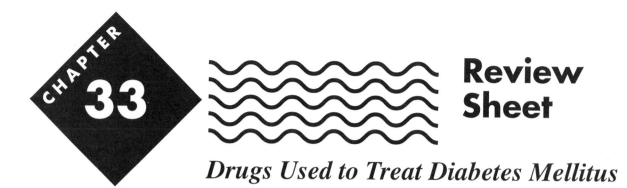

Review Sheet

Drugs Used to Treat Diabetes Mellitus

The QUESTION column and the ANSWER column have been offset so that you can cover the answers while reading the questions, allowing you to assess your knowledge.

Question

1. Diabetes mellitus is a disease that causes abnormal metabolism of _____.
2. "Insulin-dependent diabetes" (formerly IDDM) is now known as _____.
3. "Type 2 diabetes" was formerly known as _____.
4. "Gestational diabetes" (GDM) is _____.
5. "Hypoglycemia" is _____.
6. "Hyperglycemia" is _____.
7. "Polydipsia" is _____.
8. "Polyuria" is _____.
9. What are the symptoms of neuropathies?
10. What is the immediate goal for treatment of diabetes mellitus?
11. What does the treatment of type 2 diabetes mellitus require?
12. What does the treatment of type 1 diabetes mellitus require?
13. The dietary prescription for a person with diabetes mellitus, according to the American Diabetic Association (ADA), should be composed of _____% carbohydrates, _____% fats, and _____% proteins.
14. What are the recommended guidelines for glucose levels while exercising?
15. What are the usual causes of hypoglycemia?
16. When should ketone testing of the urine be performed?

Answer

1. Fats, proteins, and carbohydrates.
2. Type 1 diabetes mellitus.
3. Noninsulin-dependent diabetes mellitus (NIDDM).
4. The development of an abnormal glucose tolerance in pregnant women.
5. Low blood sugar.
6. High blood sugar.
7. Increased thirst.
8. Increased frequency of urination.
9. Numbness and tingling of extremities (paresthesia), loss of sensations, postural hypotension, impotence, and difficulty controlling urination.
10. Prevent ketoacidosis and symptoms resulting from hyperglycemia.
11. Adequate weight reduction, dietary control, and possibly the use of oral hypoglycemic or antihyperglycemic agents.
12. Adequate weight reduction, dietary control, and use of exogenous insulin.
13. 50% to 60% carbohydrates, 30% fats (primarily polyunsaturated), and 10-20% proteins (0.8 g protein/kg body weight). High-fiber foods and low sodium, alcohol, and caffeine consumption are also advisable.
14. Individuals should not exercise with glucose level above 250 mg/dl or less than 100 mg/dl.
15. Too much insulin, insufficient food intake to cover insulin taken, imbalances from diarrhea and vomiting, or excessive exercise without additional carbohydrate intake are common causes of hypoglycemia.

Copyright © 2001 by Mosby, Inc. All rights reserved.

17. What is the difference between the glycosylated hemoglobin and fructosamine tests to measure glucose?
18. What signs and symptoms result from peripheral vascular disease?

19. What types of visual complications are persons with diabetes mellitus more susceptible to?

20. How often should persons with diabetes mellitus have an eye exam?

21. How can complications of diabetes affecting the kidneys be identified?

22. What is the source of endogenous insulin? What are the primary animal sources of exogenous insulins?

23. What methods are used to produce human exogenous insulin?

24. Why are allergic reactions to regular insulin and semilente and lente Iletin I and II more common than with Humulin and Novolin forms of insulin?
25. Why can't insulin be administered orally?

26. Differentiate among *onset, peak*, and *duration* in relation to insulin therapy.
27. What is the most rapid-acting form of insulin manufactured today?

28. Do exogenous insulins differ in terms of onset, peak, and duration of action?
29. What does "U-100" mean?
30. What kind of syringe is used to measure U-100 insulin?
31. What is the only type of insulin used intravenously?

32. Why is it important to teach the patient to rotate insulin sites within one area before proceeding to the next area on a rotation schedule?

16. When serum glucose is 240 mg/dl or above, test for the presence of ketones.

17. The glycosylated hemoglobin measures glucose control over the previous 8 to 10 weeks, while the fructosamine test measures the amount of glucose bonded to the protein fructosamine over the previous 1 to 3 weeks. Each has a benefit in measuring glucose control.
18. Cyanosis or reddish-blue discoloration in the hands, feet, and legs. Pallor and coolness in the feet and legs. Ulcerations may develop. When any circulatory impairment is found, pedal and radial pulses should be checked at least every 4 hours.
19. Blurred vision may occur with hyperglycemia. With advanced diabetes mellitus, there are changes in small blood vessels in the eyes (microangiopathies). Retinal hemorrhages, degeneration of retinal vascular tissue, cataracts, and blindness may also occur.
20. Regular eye exams to detect changes in the eye should be performed at least annually and more often as deemed appropriate by the physician.
21. Presence of proteinuria, elevated serum creatinine, and blood urea nitrogen. Persons with diabetes mellitus are more likely to have urinary tract infections.
22. Endogenous insulin is produced by the beta cells of the pancreas. Synthetic insulin is the primary source of insulin for recently diagnosed diabetics. Beef and pork pancreases are the primary animal sources of exogenous insulin, but fish and sheep pancreases have been used as well.
23. Most common source of human insulin production is with recombinant DNA.

24. Humulin and Novalin insulin are manufactured synthetically, whereas the other forms of insulin listed are animal proteins (beef or pork).
25. Insulin is destroyed by the proteolytic enzymes in the gastrointestinal tract.
26. Onset is the time required for the initial effect of insulin to occur. Peak is the time of the maximum effect of insulin. Duration is the length of time insulin remains active.
27. Insulin analog injection Humalog (lispro) onset: 0.25 hr; peak: 0.5-1.5 hr; duration: 6-8 hrs.
28. Yes. See Table 33-2, p. 440.
29. U-100 means 100 units of insulin are contained in 1 ml of solution.
30. An insulin syringe calibrated in 100 units has been available for years; however, because U-100 = 100 units in 1 ml, a tuberculin syringe could also be used to accurately measure the dosage.
31. Regular insulin

Copyright © 2001 by Mosby, Inc. All rights reserved.

33. What effect does the long-term use of one injection site have on insulin absorption?
34. With increased activity and exercise, what adjustment may be required in the insulin dose?

35. When are patients who are receiving fast-acting, intermediate-acting, or extended-acting insulin most likely to develop hypoglycemia if the dose is excessive or meals are not taken as planned?
36. When are blood or urine tests for glucose performed in relation to meals and insulin administration?

37. Differentiate between the symptoms of hypoglycemia and hyperglycemia.
38. What are the treatments for hypoglycemia and hyperglycemia?

39. If uncertain whether a patient is hypoglycemic or hyperglycemic, what action should be taken?

40. What complications are associated with diabetes mellitus?
41. Describe the procedure for mixing two insulins in the same syringe.

42. At what temperature should insulin be prior to administration?
43. What types of insulin can be mixed in the same syringe and stored for use at a later time (e.g., 1 to 2 weeks later) rather than used immediately?
44. What effect does the administration of beta-adrenergic blocking agents concurrent with insulin have on symptoms of hypoglycemia?

45. What drug class does the drug metformin (Glucophage) belong to and what is its mechanism of action compared to oral sulfonylureas?

32. To prevent hypertrophy or atrophy of subcutaneous tissue.
33. Absorption is prolonged and control of glucose may require an increase in the insulin dose. If switching from an injection site that has been used repeatedly to one used infrequently, the dose of insulin may need to be decreased to prevent hypoglycemia. Each patient is somewhat variable, but patients may become hypoglycemic. A snack may be required to cover the action of the insulin, or the insulin dose could be reduced if the increased activity can be anticipated.
34. Because of risk of hypoglycemia, the insulin dose could be reduced if increased activity can be anticipated.

35. If the patient injects insulin at 7 AM, fast-acting insulin may induce hypoglycemia before lunch; intermediate-acting insulin between 3 PM and dinner; and extended-acting insulin between 2 AM and breakfast.
36. 1/2 hour ac and hs

37. Hypoglycemia: rapid onset, nervousness, tremors, headache, apprehension, sweating, hunger, double or blurred vision, lack of coordination, unconsciousness
Hyperglycemia: gradual onset, increased thirst, headache, nausea and vomiting, rapid pulse, shallow respirations, acetone odor on breath, unconsciousness
38. Hypoglycemia: If conscious and able to swallow: 2-4 oz fruit juice with 2 teaspoons sugar or honey added, or 1 cup skim milk, 4 oz nondiet soft drink, or piece of candy (not chocolate), or frosting added. If unable to swallow: 20 to 50 ml glucose 50% IV.
Hyperglycemia: Hospitalize patient, identify the cause, hydrate the patient and give insulin IV; stabilize electrolytes, especially potassium.
See also drug monograph for glucagon.
39. Treat for hypoglycemia.

40. Peripheral vascular disease, renal vascular disease, increased frequency of infections, progressive blindness, neuropathies.
41. See Figure 9-23, Chapter 9: Parenteral Administration.
42. Room temperature (Refrigerate, do not freeze, extra vials of insulin.)

43. Table 33-3: Regular and NPH can be mixed and stored for up to 2 to 3 months. Regular and lente combinations may be mixed but should be used immediately. Any combination of lentes are stable indefinitely.
44. Beta adrenergic blocking agents mask the signs of hypoglycemia.

 Copyright © 2001 by Mosby, Inc. All rights reserved.

46. How do oral hypoglycemic agents differ from insulin?

47. Which type of diabetes mellitus requires treatment with insulin and which type may be treated with oral hypoglycemic agents?

48. For what type of allergy should you check the chart and the patient before initiating therapy with an oral sulfonylurea hypoglycemic agent?

49. What is the effect of sulfonylurea hypoglycemic agents combined with ethanol on blood glucose levels?

50. When should a diabetic patient perform urine testing for ketones?

51. What are the therapeutic outcomes expected from a biguanide oral hypoglycemic agent?

52. What is the mechanism of action of meglitinide oral hypoglycemic agents and what drug belongs to this class?

53. What is the mechanism of action of the thiazolidinedione (TZD) oral hypoglycemic agents? What agents belong to this class?

54. As antihyperglycemic agents, what is the mechanism of action of acarbose (Precose) and miglitol (Glyset)?

55. What side effects can be expected with acarbose (Precose) and miglitol (Glyset)?

56. What affect can acarbose and miglitol have on digoxin absorption?

57. What is the action of glucagon?

45. Biguanide oral hypoglycemic agents—mechanism of action unknown. It does not stimulate release of insulin from the pancreas like the sulfonylureas.

46. For sulfonylurea oral hypoglycemic agents to be effective, the diabetic patient must still have beta cells in the pancreas that are capable of producing insulin. These agents act by stimulating the release of insulin from the beta cells. Oral hypoglycemic agents are not an oral form of insulin. The newer class, biguanide oral hypoglycemics [e.g., metaformin (Glucophage)], do not stimulate release of insulin from the pancreas; the mechanism of their action is unknown.

47. Type 1 diabetes mellitus uses insulin; type 2 diabetes mellitus may be treated with diet and oral hypoglycemic agents. (See specific information in text.)

48. Sulfonamides. The patient who is allergic to sulfonamides may also be allergic to sulfonylureas.

49. Hypoglycemia. Also may result in an Antabuse-like reaction manifested by facial flushing, pounding headache, breathlessness, and nausea.

50. Perform urine testing for ketones whenever the blood glucose is 240 mg/dL or above and whenever under stress or having an infection. Perform at least four times daily under these circumstances.

51. Decrease in FBS and glycosylated hemoglobin concentration and fewer long-term complications from poorly controlled type 2 diabetes.

52. Repaglinide (Prandin) is a nonsulfonylurea hypoglycemic agent that lowers the blood glucose by stimulating release of insulin from the beta cells of the pancreas.

53. Pioglitazone and rosiglitazone, known as TZDs, lower the glucose by increasing the sensitivity of muscle and fat tissue to insulin, allowing more glucose to enter the cells in the presence of insulin.

54. Acarbose and miglitol inhibit the pancreatic enzyme alpha amylase, which digests sugars in the GI tract. This results in delayed glucose absorption and lowered postprandial hyperglycemia.

55. Abdominal cramps, diarrhea, flatulence. Resolves with continued use of acarbose or miglitol.

56. These drugs may inhibit digoxin absorption.

57. Glucagon breaks down stored glycogen to glucose to be used as an energy source.

Copyright © 2001 by Mosby, Inc.   All rights reserved.

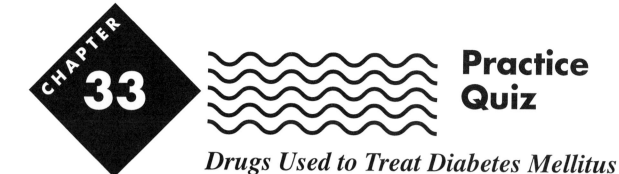

Practice Quiz

Drugs Used to Treat Diabetes Mellitus

TRUE OR FALSE

Mark "T" for true and "F" for false for each statement.
Correct all false statements.

_____ 1. Type 1 diabetes mellitus does not require insulin.

_____ 2. Exercise lowers the blood glucose level.

_____ 3. When ketones are high in a urine sample, the individual is hypoglycemic.

_____ 4. When beta cells are absent, no insulin is produced.

_____ 5. The ADA recommends 30% carbohydrates, 12 to 20% fats, and 55 to 60% proteins in a diabetic diet.

_____ 6. Ingestion of alcohol on an empty stomach may cause hyperglycemia.

_____ 7. A snack should be eaten before exercise if the blood glucose is less than 100 mg/dL.

_____ 8. Possible causes of hypoglycemia include too much insulin, extra food intake to cover insulin, and excessive exercise without a CHO snack beforehand.

_____ 9. Persons using oral hypoglycemic agents do not require any insulin.

_____ 10. Drugs known as oral sulfonylurea agents act by stimulating release of insulin from beta cells.

_____ 11. The glycosylated hemoglobin test monitors a client's glucose level over the previous 1 to 3 weeks.

_____ 12. Hyperglycemic reactions are generally of short duration and require a dose of subcutaneous insulin stat.

_____ 13. Beta adrenergic blockers given concurrently with insulin block the signs and symptoms of hyperglycemia.

_____ 14. Repaglinide (Prandin) lowers the blood glucose by stimulating the release of insulin from the beta cells of the pancreas.

_____ 15. Acarbose (Precose) is an antihyperglycemic agent that lowers glucose levels by delaying glucose absorption.

COMPLETION

Complete the following statements.

16. Treatment of hypoglycemia in a conscious, patient includes _____
_____.

17. Treatment of hyperglycemia includes _____
_____.

18. Insulin is required to transport glucose into skeletal and heart muscle and fat. It is not required for glucose transport into _____.

19. _____ type insulin may be given intravenously and subcutaneously.

20. Long-acting, suspension form of insulin is
_____.

21. Insulin should be stored _____.

22. Humalog (lispro) (can, cannot) be administered IV because it is a clear form of insulin.

END-OF-CHAPTER MATH REVIEW

1. Ordered: 22 U NPH (human) insulin to be administered 30 minutes before breakfast.
   Available: U-100 NPH (human) insulin
   Volume of insulin to be administered: _____ ml

2. Ordered: 27 U NPH (human) insulin + 7 U regular (human) insulin to be administered before breakfast.
   Available: U-100 NPH (human) insulin
   U-100 regular (human) insulin
   a. Volume of NPH insulin to be drawn up: _____ ml
   b. Volume of regular insulin to be drawn up: _____ ml
   c. Total volume to be injected: _____ ml

Copyright © 2001 by Mosby, Inc.   All rights reserved.

CRITICAL THINKING QUESTIONS

Situation: R.V., age 18, was recently diagnosed with type 1 diabetes mellitus. After several days of treatment with adjustment of diet, exercise, and regular insulin, R.V. was placed on U-100 NPH (human) insulin, 20 U 30 minutes before breakfast and 10 U before the evening meal.

1. What are the nursing interventions to be considered when administering the NPH insulin?
2. R.V. is having trouble injecting himself. In a moment of frustration, he asks, "Why can't I take insulin pills like my grandfather?" What is your response?

Five days later, the physician adds 5 U of regular (human) insulin to the morning dose to be administered with the NPH insulin.

3. Describe how you would teach R.V. to mix the morning insulin dose for a single administration.
4. While continuing with R.V.'s education, he asks again for the difference between the symptoms of hypoglycemia and hyperglycemia. What is your response?

Copyright © 2001 by Mosby, Inc. All rights reserved.

Syllabus

Drugs Used to Treat Thyroid Disease

CHAPTER CONTENTS

CHAPTER OBJECTIVES

1. Describe the signs, symptoms, treatment, and nursing interventions associated with hypothyroidism and hyperthyroidism.
2. Identify the two classes of drugs used to treat thyroid disease.
3. Name the drug of choice for hypothyroidism.
4. Explain the effects of hyperthyroidism on dosages of warfarin and digitalis glycosides and on persons taking oral hypoglycemic agents.
5. Discuss the actions of antithyroid medications on the formation and release of the hormones produced by the thyroid gland.
6. State the three types of treatment for hyperthyroidism.
7. Explain the nutritional requirements and activity restrictions needed for individuals with hyperthyroidism.
8. Identify the types of conditions that respond favorably to the use of radioactive iodine-131.
9. Explain the action of propylthiouracil on the synthesis of T_3 and T_4.

KEY WORDS

thyroid stimulating hormone
triiodothyronine (T_3)
thyroxine (T_4)
hypothyroidism
myxedema
cretinism
hyperthyroidism
thyrotoxicosis

ASSIGNMENTS

Read textbook pp. 450-458.
Study Key Words associated with chapter content.
Study Review Sheet for Chapter 34.
Complete End-of-Chapter Math Review and Critical Thinking Questions.
Complete Collaborative Activities as assigned by instructor.
Complete Chapter 34 Practice Quiz.
Complete Chapter 34 Exam.

COLLABORATIVE ACTIVITIES

Complete the following as preparation for in-class discussion and group work that may be assigned by the instructor.

1. Research the hospital policy for management of radioactive spills.
2. Research the hospital guidelines/policy for handling patient excreta following the administration of I^{131}.

Copyright © 2001 by Mosby, Inc.   All rights reserved.

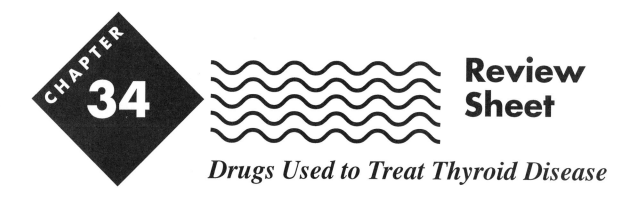

CHAPTER 34

Review Sheet

Drugs Used to Treat Thyroid Disease

The QUESTION column and the ANSWER column have been offset so that you can cover the answers while reading the questions, allowing you to assess your knowledge.

Question

1. What glands regulate the function of the thyroid gland?
2. What body functions are regulated by the thyroid gland?
3. What is another name for myxedema?

4. Excessive thyroid secretion results in what conditions?
5. What is a normal thyroid state called?
6. Thyroid replacement hormones are used to replace what hormones secreted by the thyroid gland?
7. What focused assessment should be performed by the nurse when a patient has hypothyroid or hyperthyroid disorders?
8. If a patient has hypothyroidism, what change in his or her weight over the past few months could be anticipated?
9. A patient with hyperthyroidism may require what dietary changes?
10. What type of environment does a patient with hypothyroidism or hyperthyroidism need?
11. List the thyroid hormone replacement products' brand names and ingredients.
12. Of the thyroid products available, which has the most rapid onset of action?

13. Are thyroid replacement hormones given to a patient with hypothyroidism or hyperthyroidism?
14. List the signs and symptoms of hypothyroidism and hyperthyroidism.
15. What are the three products available to treat hyperthyroidism?

Answer

1. Hypothalamus and anterior pituitary gland

2. Growth and maturation; carbohydrate, protein, and lipid metabolism; thermal regulation; cardiovascular function; lactation; and reproduction are all functions affected by thyroid function.
3. Hypothyroidism in adult patients.

4. Hyperthyroidism, also known as thyrotoxicosis.
5. Euthyroid state

6. Liothyronine (T_3) and levothyroxine (T_4)

7. See textbook pp. 451-452.

8. Weight gain

9. Increase in calories to meet metabolic needs—as much as 4000 to 5000 calories daily.
10. Hypothyroidism = warm environment
    hyperthyroidism = cool environment
11. Levothyroxine (T_4)—(Synthroid, Levoxyl)
    Liothyronine (T_3)—(Cytomel)
    Liotrix (T_3, T_4)—(Thyrolar)
    Thyroid USP
12. Liothyronine (T_3) (Cytomel)

13. Hypothyroidism

14. See textbook pp. 450-451.

Copyright © 2001 by Mosby, Inc. All rights reserved.

16. State the action of propylthiouracil (PTU) and methimazole.
17. Describe the desired therapeutic outcome(s) for antithyroid medications.

18. What are the side effects to assess when propylthiouracil or methimazole are administered?

19. What laboratory studies should be performed at periodic intervals for people taking propylthiouracil?

20. Would a patient with hyperthyroidism be more likely to require a smaller or larger dose of a digitalis glycoside?

15. Radioactive iodine (I^{131}), propylthiouracil (PTU, Propacil), and methimazole (Tapazole)
16. Propylthiouracil (PTU) and methimazole block the synthesis of T_3 and T_4 in the thyroid gland; the drugs do not destroy T_3 and T_4 already produced.
17. The primary therapeutic outcome expected from propylthiouracil or methimazole is a gradual return to normal thyroid metabolic function.
18. Skin eruptions, pruritus, headaches, salivary or lymph node enlargement, sore throat, purpura, jaundice, and progressive weakness
19. RBC, WBC, and differential counts

20. A larger dose

Copyright © 2001 by Mosby, Inc. All rights reserved.

Practice Quiz

Drugs Used to Treat Thyroid Disease

TRUE OR FALSE

Mark "T" for true and "F" for false. <u>*Correct all false statements.*</u>

_____ 1. Hyperthyroidism is a condition caused by excessive production of thyroid hormone.

_____ 2. Thyroid replacement hormones block the release of T_3 and T_4 in the body, thereby making the hormones available for metabolic functioning.

_____ 3. Baseline premedication assessments prior to initiation of thyroid replacement hormones are vital signs, weight, bowel elimination pattern, and laboratory studies to identify thyroid hormone levels.

_____ 4. The hypothyroid patient will be hyperactive.

_____ 5. The resting pulse rate of a hyperthyroid patient upon awakening will be low.

_____ 6. A patient with hypothyroidism would show dramatic weight loss as one of their symptoms.

ESSAY

7. List the signs and symptoms of hypothyroidism and hyperthyroidism. When thyroid replacement hormones are administered, how should these signs and symptoms be monitored?

END-OF-CHAPTER MATH REVIEW

1. Ordered: Levothyroxine (Synthroid) 0.1 mg po daily
   On hand: Levothyroxine (Synthroid) 0.05 mg tablets
   Give: _____ tablets.

2. Ordered: Levothyroxine (Synthroid) 200 mcg
   Convert 200 mcg to mg.
   _____ mg

CRITICAL THINKING QUESTIONS

Situation: J.T.'s baseline vital signs are BP 140/60, pulse 104, respirations 24. He has been receiving levothyroxine (Synthroid) 0.1 mg po daily for the past six weeks for treatment of hypothyroidism.

He reports that his resting pulse on awakening has been 90-112 over the past week.

1. Should these findings be reported to the physician?

2. If so, what additional data should be assembled before initiating physician contact?

Situation: S.G. is taking propylthiouracil 50 mg po tid.

1. What patient education should be provided to her regarding side effects to expect and side effects to report?

Copyright © 2001 by Mosby, Inc.   All rights reserved.

CHAPTER 35

Corticosteroids

CHAPTER CONTENTS

Corticosteroids (p. 458)
Drug Therapy: Corticosteroids (p. 461)
    Drug Class: Mineralocorticoids (p. 461)
    Drug Class: Glucocorticoids (p. 463)

CHAPTER OBJECTIVES

1. Review the functions of the adrenal gland.
2. State the normal actions of mineralocorticoids and glucocorticoids in the body.
3. Cite the disease states caused by hypersecretion or hyposecretion of the adrenal gland.
4. Identify the baseline assessments needed for a patient receiving corticosteroids.
5. Prepare a list of the clinical uses of mineralocorticoids and glucocorticoids.
6. Discuss the potential side effects associated with the use of corticosteroids and give examples of specific patient education needed for patients taking these agents.
7. Develop measurable objectives for patient education for persons taking corticosteroids.

KEY WORDS

corticosteroids
mineralocorticoids
glucocorticoids
cortisol

ASSIGNMENTS

Read textbook pp. 458-465.
Study Key Words associated with chapter content.
Study Review Sheet for Chapter 35.
Complete End-of-Chapter Math Review and Critical Thinking Questions.
Complete Collaborative Activity as assigned by instructor.
Complete Chapter 35 Practice Quiz.
Complete Chapter 35 Exam.

COLLABORATIVE ACTIVITY

Complete the following as preparation for in-class discussion and group work that may be assigned by the instructor.

Develop a patient education plan for an individual with a glucocorticoid prescribed for treatment of rheumatoid arthritis. (Use drug monograph and other resources.)

Copyright © 2001 by Mosby, Inc.   All rights reserved.

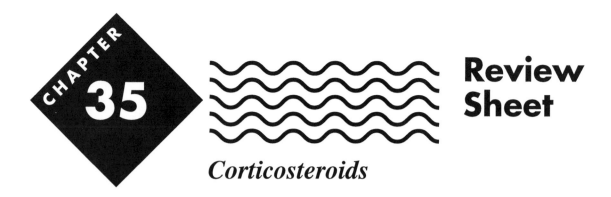

Review Sheet

Corticosteroids

The QUESTION column and the ANSWER column have been offset so that you can cover the answers while reading the questions, allowing you to assess your knowledge.

Question	**Answer**
1. Define *corticosteroids*.	1. Hormones secreted by the adrenal cortex of the adrenal gland.
2. For what types of illnesses are glucocorticoids frequently prescribed?	2. To treat diseases or disorders that are inflammatory or allergic in nature.
3. What endogenous hormone is known as a glucocorticoid?	3. Cortisol
4. Do exogenous corticosteroids cure disease?	4. Exogenous corticosteroids do not cure disease unless the adrenal glands have been surgically removed and corticosteroids are used for replacement therapy. Usually, steroids provide relief of symptoms without treating the underlying disease.
5. What side effects may be observed with the administration of glucocorticoids?	5. Hyperglycemia, glycosuria (corticosteroids stimulate formation of glucose while decreasing use of glucose by the body); electrolyte imbalances and fluid accumulation due to mineralocorticoid effects that cause sodium and water retention and potassium and hydrogen excretion; increased susceptibility to infection; peptic ulcer formation by decreasing the protective secretions of the gastric mucosa; delayed wound healing because of protein breakdown; visual changes, cataracts; osteoporosis—inhibits bone formation and growth; see textbook pp. 463, 465.
6. What time of day is best to administer glucocorticoids?	6. Between 6 AM and 9 AM to minimize suppression of normal adrenal function.
7. Why do corticosteroids and diuretics produce or enhance hypokalemia when given simultaneously?	7. Diuretics (except potassium-sparing diuretics) and corticosteroids cause the loss of potassium.
8. Why must patients taking corticosteroids be cautioned to avoid contact with persons with infections?	8. Corticosteroids diminish the production of antibodies, resulting in a suppressed immune system, making the patient susceptible to infection. The anti-inflammatory properties of these drugs also mask the presence of infection. Even the slightest signs and symptoms of an infection may indicate the presence of a major infection.
9. What instructions should be given to a patient taking corticosteroids?	9. See textbook pp. 460-461.
10. What baseline assessments should be completed for patients taking any type of corticosteroids?	

 Copyright © 2001 by Mosby, Inc. All rights reserved.

11. Review the signs and symptoms of Addison's disease and Cushing's disease and contrast these with the signs and symptoms of adrenocortical excess and deficiency.

12. What effect do glucocorticoids have on blood glucose levels?

13. What type of health teaching should be done for a client receiving steroid therapy?

14. What is the major glucocorticoid secreted by the adrenal cortex?

15. Why is an alternate day schedule for administration of corticosteroids used?

16. What effect do corticosteroids have on potassium balance?

10. Daily weight; blood pressure in supine and sitting position; intake and output for hospitalized patients; electrolyte studies, especially sodium and potassium; check mental status; blood glucose; signs and symptoms of infection; signs and symptoms of ulcers.

11. See a general medical/surgical nursing text.

12. Hyperglycemia.

13. Identification bracelet, *do not* suddenly discontinue drug therapy. See textbook for specific drug therapy prescribed by reviewing the drug monograph.

14. Cortisol

15. Alternate day schedule, between 6 AM and 9 AM, minimizes suppression of normal adrenal function. Also administer with meals to minimize gastric irritation.

16. Enhance loss of potassium. Be especially alert when diuretics such as furosemide, thiazides, bumetanide, and other non-potassium–sparing diuretics are prescribed concurrently.

Copyright © 2001 by Mosby, Inc.   All rights reserved.

Corticosteroids

Practice Quiz

TRUE OR FALSE

Mark "T" for true and "F" for false. <u>*Correct all false*</u>
<u>*statements.*</u>

_____ 1. Corticosteroids are secreted from the adrenal medulla.

_____ 2. Psychotic behavior may be seen during corticosteroid therapy.

_____ 3. Individuals receiving glucocorticoid therapy should be monitored for hyperglycemia if they are diabetic or prediabetic.

_____ 4. Glucocorticoids taken for long-term therapy may produce cataracts.

_____ 5. Corticosteroid therapy does not mask the signs and symptoms of infection.

_____ 6. To minimize suppression of normal adrenal function corticosteroids may be administered on alternate days.

_____ 7. Corticosteroids should not be discontinued abruptly.

_____ 8. Glucocorticoids should be administered between 6 PM and 9 PM to maintain normal adrenal function.

_____ 9. The major glucocorticoid secreted by the adrenal cortex is cortisol.

END-OF-CHAPTER MATH REVIEW

1. The package insert accompanying prednisone states that the physiologic replacement (pediatric) is 0.1–0.15 mg/kg/day, po, in equal divided doses q 12 h. The child's weight is 22 lbs.
   22 lbs. equals _____kg.

2. Using the dosage parameters described above, calculate the minimum and maximum dose per day for this child's weight.
   _____ mg minimum
   _____ mg maximum

CRITICAL THINKING QUESTIONS

1. C.L. is receiving prednisone for treatment of hypercalcemia associated with cancer. He tells you, with great excitement, that his young grandchildren are coming to stay at his home for the next several months. What precautions should be taught to him and immediate family members regarding exposure to the grandchildren, especially when the children receive pediatric immunizations?

2. What data would indicate a positive clinical response following the administration of adrenal cortical hormones prescribed for the treatment of Addison's disease?

Copyright © 2001 by Mosby, Inc.   All rights reserved.

Syllabus

Gonadal Hormones

CHAPTER CONTENTS

The Gonads and Gonadal Hormones (p. 466)
Drug Therapy with Gonadal Hormones (p. 467)
    Drug Class: Estrogens (p. 467)
    Drug Class: Progestins (p. 468)
    Drug Class: Androgens (p. 468)

CHAPTER OBJECTIVES

1. Describe the body changes that can be anticipated with the administration of androgens, estrogens, or progesterone.
2. State the uses of estrogens and progestins.
3. Compare the side effects of estrogen hormones with those of a combination of estrogen and progesterone.
4. Differentiate between the side effects to expect and side effects to report with the administration of estrogen or progesterone.
5. Identify the rationale for administering androgens to women who have certain types of breast cancer.

KEY WORDS

gonads
testes
ovaries
testosterone

androgens
estrogen
progesterone

ASSIGNMENTS

Read textbook pp. 466-472.
Study Key Words associated with chapter content.
Study Review Sheet for Chapter 36.
Complete End-of-Chapter Math Review and Critical Thinking Questions.
Complete Collaborative Activity as assigned by instructor.
Complete Chapter 36 Practice Quiz.
Complete Chapter 36 Exam.

COLLABORATIVE ACTIVITY

Complete the following as preparation for in-class discussion and group work that may be assigned by the instructor.

Explain the rationale for administering androgens to women with certain types of breast cancer.

Copyright © 2001 by Mosby, Inc.   All rights reserved.

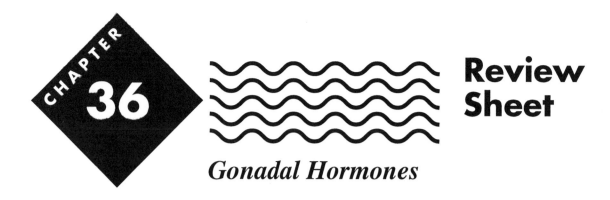

Review Sheet

Gonadal Hormones

The QUESTION column and the ANSWER column have been offset so that you can cover the answers while reading the questions, allowing you to assess your knowledge.

Question

1. What is another name for the male sex hormones?
2. What male characteristics are attributed to androgens?
3. When androgens are given to females, what effects can be anticipated?

4. Describe the effect of the administration of testosterone to boys before completion of bone growth.

5. When would androgens be prescribed for females?

6. Why is testosterone derived naturally from animal testes not administered orally?

7. What type of testosterone can be administered orally?
8. Review the uses and effects of estrogens on the body systems.
9. What are the side effects to expect and those to report for persons taking estrogen products?
10. What are progestins used to treat?

11. What happens to the progesterone level if fertilization does not take place?

12. What premedication assessments should be performed prior to therapy with estrogens, progestins, and androgens?
13. What effect can androgen therapy have on calcium in patients being treated for breast cancer?

Answer

1. Androgens; testosterone is the primary hormone.

2. Normal growth and development of male sex organs and secondary sex characteristics (e.g., growth and maturation of prostate, seminal vesicles, penis, and scrotum; development and distribution of male hair on the body; deepening of the voice).

3. Masculinization, if given in sufficient doses (e.g., deepening voice, hirsutism, acne, menstrual irregularity); electrolyte imbalance of Na^+, K^+, Cl^- and Ca^{++}; gastric irritation.

4. May cause premature closure of the epiphyseal line, inhibiting normal bone growth.

5. In some types of breast cancer and to prevent lactation and breast engorgement in the nonnursing mother.

6. It is rapidly inactivated by the liver.

7. Synthetic forms (e.g., methyltestosterone, fluoxymesterone)

8. See textbook, p. 467.

9. Expect: weight gain, edema, breast tenderness, nausea. Report: hypertension, hyperglycemia, thrombophlebitis, breakthrough vaginal bleeding.

10. Secondary amenorrhea, breakthrough bleeding, endometriosis, and when combined with estrogen, used as an oral contraceptive.

11. Progesterone production drops and menstruation occurs.

12. See textbook: estrogens, p. 468; progestins, p. 468; androgens, p. 470.

13. Hypercalcemia

Copyright © 2001 by Mosby, Inc.   All rights reserved.

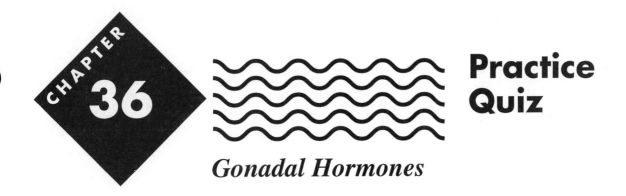

Practice Quiz

Gonadal Hormones

COMPLETION

Complete the following statements.

The gonads are called:

1. _____ in males
2. _____ in females

Progesterones' major body functions include:

3. _____
4. _____
5. _____

Premedication assessment before initiation of estrogen therapy should include:

6. _____
7. _____
8. _____
9. and any history of:

Progestins prevent:

10. _____
11. _____
12. Androgen therapy in females produces
    _____.

END-OF-CHAPTER MATH REVIEW

1. Ordered: Hydroxyprogesterone 375 mg IM.
   On hand: Hydroxyprogesterone 250 mg/ml
   Give: _____ ml.
2. Ordered: Progesterone 10 mg IM, daily times 6 days.
   On hand: Progesterone 50 mg/ml
   Give: _____ ml daily

CRITICAL THINKING QUESTION

S.A., age 62, is receiving methyltestosterone 200 mg po daily for palliation of breast cancer. She asks you why she is taking this particular medication and expresses concern that this, like other medications she has taken for treatment of the cancer, will make her feel ill. What should you tell her?

Copyright © 2001 by Mosby, Inc.   All rights reserved.

CHAPTER 37

Syllabus

Drugs Used in Obstetrics

CHAPTER CONTENTS

CHAPTER OBJECTIVES

1. Describe nursing assessments and nursing interventions needed for the pregnant patient during the first, second, and third trimesters of pregnancy.
2. Identify appropriate nursing assessments, nursing interventions, and treatment options used for the following obstetric complications: infection, hyperemesis gravidarum, miscarriage, abortion, preterm labor, premature rupture of membranes, gestational diabetes, and pregnancy-induced hypertension (PIH).
3. State the methods and time parameters of each approach to the termination of a pregnancy.
4. Summarize the care needs of the pregnant woman during labor and delivery and the immediate postpartum period including the patient education needed before discharge to promote safe self-care and care of the newborn.
5. State the purpose of administering glucocorticoids to certain women in preterm labor.
6. State the actions, primary uses, nursing assessments and monitoring parameters for uterine stimulants, uterine relaxants, clomiphene citrate, magnesium sulfate, and $Rh_o(D)$ immune globulin.
7. Compare the effects of uterine stimulants and uterine relaxants on the pregnant woman's uterus.
8. Describe specific nursing concerns and appropriate nursing actions when uterine stimulants are administered for induction of labor, augmentation of labor, and postpartum atony and hemorrhage.
9. Cite the effects of adrenergic agents on $beta_1$ and $beta_2$ receptors and identify the relationship of these actions to the side effects to report when adrenergic agents are used to inhibit preterm labor.

10. Describe specific assessments needed before and during the use of ritodrine, terbutaline, or magnesium sulfate.
11. Identify emergency supplies that should be available in the immediate vicinity during magnesium sulfate therapy.
12. Identify the action, specific dosage, administration precautions, and proper timing of the administration of $Rh_o(D)$ immune globulin and rubella vaccine in relation to pregnancy.
13. Summarize the immediate nursing care needs of the newborn infant following delivery.

KEY WORDS

pregnancy-induced hypertension
lochia
precipitous labor and delivery
augmentation
dysfunctional labor

ASSIGNMENTS

Read textbook pp. 473-492.
Study Key Words associated with chapter content.
Study Review Sheet for Chapter 37.
Complete End-of-Chapter Math Review and Critical Thinking Questions.
Complete Collaborative Activities as assigned by instructor.
Complete Chapter 37 Practice Quiz.
Complete Chapter 37 Exam.

COLLABORATIVE ACTIVITIES

Complete the following as preparation for in-class discussion and group work that may be assigned by the instructor.
1. Research the hospital policy for administration of oxytocin.
2. Prepare a detailed listing of nursing interventions needed during IV infusion of oxytocin.

Copyright © 2001 by Mosby, Inc.   All rights reserved.

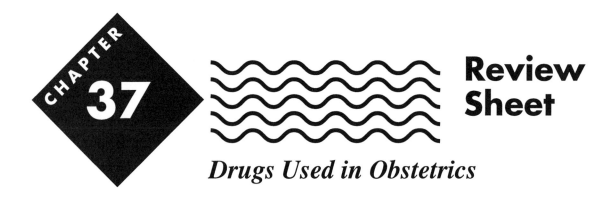

Drugs Used in Obstetrics

The QUESTION column and the ANSWER column have been offset so that you can cover the answers while reading the questions, allowing you to assess your knowledge.

Question	Answer
1. Identify the factors that need to be assessed during prenatal management of a pregnant woman and during and following normal labor and delivery.	
2. Describe nursing assessments and interventions needed for the pregnant patient experiencing potential obstetrical complications (e.g., infection; hyperemesis gravidarum; miscarriage; abortion; pregnancy-induced hypertension (PIH); hemolysis, elevated liver enzymes, low platelet syndrome (HELLP); and bleeding disorders).	1. See textbook pp. 474-475.
3. State the methods and time parameters of each approach to the termination of a pregnancy.	2. See text for details of the following categories: miscarriage, placental separation and abortion, PIH, HELLP, etc.
4. Cite the recommended times of administration for $Rh_o(D)$ immune globulin (human) and rubella vaccine in relation to pregnancy.	3. Before 12 weeks gestation: dilatation and evacuation (D&E). 12 to 20 weeks gestation: saline or prostaglandin administered intra-amniotically, intramuscularly, or by vaginal suppository. Intrauterine fetal death after 20 weeks gestation: prostaglandin suppositories with or without oxytocin augmentation.
5. Identify the signs, symptoms, and management of PIH.	4. An Rh(-) mother may receive RhoGAM within 72 hours of termination of pregnancy. Rubella vaccine should be given to a patient whose rubella titer is low, immediately after pregnancy. She should be counseled to use birth control for at least the next 3 months.
6. Describe the nursing assessments and interventions used for PIH.	5. Signs and symptoms of PIH are hypertension, edema, and proteinuria. It occurs in 5% to 7% of all pregnancies. PIH is observed most often in the last 10 weeks of gestation, during labor, and in the first 12 to 48 hours after delivery. The etiology is unknown and the only cure is termination of pregnancy.
7. State the purpose of administering glucocorticoids to certain women in preterm labor.	6. Take vital signs at regularly scheduled intervals and compare with baseline readings. Report elevations of systolic pressure of 30 mmHg or more above the previous readings, or systolic blood pressure of 140

Copyright © 2001 by Mosby, Inc. All rights reserved.

mmHg or more, or diastolic pressure of 90 mmHg or more. Edema may be present: Do I/Os and check state of hydration. Intake of 1000 ml more than the output over the preceding 24 hours is generally allowed. Perform assessment of edema: Daily weights, report a weight gain of 2 or more pounds in any one-week period. Discourage the heavy use of salt. Monitor urine for the presence of protein. Electrolyte studies should be done at regular intervals. Hematocrit will become elevated as the patient becomes dehydrated. Information from the serum estriols and L/S ratio give indications of fetal maturity. Seizure precautions: Monitor for drowsiness, hyperflexia, visual disturbances, or severe pain. Report any of these symptoms immediately! Give prescribed medications (e.g., sedatives, antihypertensives, anticonvulsants). Observe for complications (e.g., started labor, pulmonary edema, heart failure).

8. Summarize the care needs of the pregnant woman during normal labor and delivery.

9. Identify the name, dosage, route of administration, and correct time for administering oxytocic agents.
10. Describe the normal sequence of changes in the appearance of lochia during the postpartum period.
11. Summarize the immediate nursing care needs of the newborn infant following delivery.
12. Discuss the rationale for inspection of the placenta and cord following delivery of the newborn.

13. Summarize the Centers for Disease Control recommendations for prophylaxis of ophthalmia neonatorum.
14. Identify assessment data that is essential in detecting postpartum hemorrhage.

15. State the drug actions and nursing assessments needed to monitor therapeutic response and development of side effects to expect or report from uterine stimulants, uterine relaxants, clomiphene citrate, magnesium sulfate, $Rh_o(D)$ immune globulin, and erythromycin ophthalmic ointment.
16. List premedication assessments needed prior to an oxytocin infusion.
17. What are signs and symptoms of fetal distress?

7. Glucocorticoids are administered IM to the woman in preterm labor to accelerate fetal lung maturation and to minimize hyaline membrane disease.
8. See textbook pp. 478-479 for summary of normal labor and delivery needs.
9. See textbook pp. 485-486 for a discussion of oxytocic agents.

10. Blood red immediately after delivery, progressing to a more watery or pinkish color.
11. See text discussion: Assessment of the Neonate, p. 475.
12. Verify presence of one vein and two arteries in the cord and inspect the placenta to be certain it is intact and no fragments or pieces have been retained.
13. See textbook p. 479 for acceptable agents that prevent gonococcal ophthalmia neonatorum and chlamydial ophthalmia neonatorum.
14. Fundus height and firmness. Lochia color and amount. Vital signs.

15. See individual drug monographs for details.

16. Maternal vital signs, especially blood pressure; mother's hydration status including urine output and I & O. (This will form baseline data for subsequent monitoring during drug therapy.) Monitor characteristics of uterine contractions (e.g., frequency, rate, duration and intensity); report duration over 90 seconds. Monitor fetal heart rate and rhythm. Perform reflex testing as specified in drug monograph. Check amount and characteristics of vaginal discharge.

Copyright © 2001 by Mosby, Inc. All rights reserved.

18. If fetal distress occurs during oxytocin therapy, what actions should be taken immediately?
19. State the primary clinical indications for use of uterine stimulants.

20. Describe specific nursing concerns and appropriate nursing actions when uterine stimulants are administered for induction of labor, augmentation of labor, and postpartum atony and hemorrhage.

21. Explain the limitations of the use of oxytocin for the purpose of initiating a therapeutic abortion.

22. Review the procedure for insertion of vaginal suppositories.
23. Differentiate among the uses and actions on the uterus of dinoprostone, ergonovine maleate, methylergonovine maleate, and oxytocin.
24. Identify specific nursing assessments, interventions, and evaluation criteria used during the administration of uterine stimulants.

25. Compare the effects of methylergonovine maleate and ergonovine maleate on lactation.
26. Identify specific actions, dosage and administration, and nursing assessments needed during the use of oxytocin therapy.
27. What is the effect of oxytocin on fluid balance?

17. Normal fetal heart rate (120 to 160 beats/min.); report bradycardia (below 120) tachycardia (over 160).
18. Slow oxytocin infusion to lowest rate in accordance with hospital policy. Turn mother to left lateral position, administer O_2 by mask or cannula, call the physician immediately.
19. Four primary clinical uses: (1) induction or augmentation of labor; (2) control of postpartum atony and hemorrhage; (3) control of postsurgical hemorrhage (e.g., C-section); and (4) induction of therapeutic abortion.
20. Induction of labor: Check vital signs q 15 minutes, use an infusion pump, monitor contractions (e.g., frequency, duration, and intensity), and fetal heart tones. Monitor for fetal distress (fetal heart rate of 160 bpm followed by bradycardia below 120 bpm). If fetal distress occurs, reduce oxytocin infusion to the slowest rate, turn mother to left lateral position, and administer oxygen. Monitor the intake and output of all patients receiving oxytocin and report accumulation of water by the body, known as "water intoxication."
21. Uterine smooth muscle is not very responsive to oxytocin stimulation until late in the third trimester.
22. See Administration of Vaginal Medications (pp. 153-154).

23. Dinoprostone: Uterine smooth muscle stimulant. Used during pregnancy to increase the frequency and strength of uterine contractions and produce cervical softening and dilatation. Used to expel uterine contents in cases of intrauterine fetal death, benign hydatidiform mole, missed spontaneous miscarriage, and second trimester abortion. Ergonovine maleate, methylergonovine maleate: Both stimulate contractions of the uterus. Cannot be used for induction of labor because they cause sudden intense uterine activity. Used in postpartum patients to control bleeding and maintain uterine firmness. Oxytocin: Stimulates smooth muscle of the uterus, blood vessels, and mammary glands. Can be used during the third trimester to initiate labor. Drug of choice to induce labor at term or to augment uterine contractions during first and second stages of labor.
24. See number 20 above.

25. Do not use ergonovine in patients who wish to breastfeed. Methylergonovine may be used.

26. Observe the rate of infusion of oxytocin and the fetal monitor for measurement of contractions. Assess for nausea, vomiting, fetal distress, hypertension or hypotension, seizure activity, and water intoxication.

Copyright © 2001 by Mosby, Inc. All rights reserved.

28. Compare the effects of uterine stimulants and uterine relaxants on the pregnant uterus.

29. Review the effects of adrenergic agents on beta$_1$ and beta$_2$ receptors and identify the relationship of these actions to the side effects to report when adrenergic agents are used to inhibit preterm labor.
30. What are the effects of adrenergic agents on serum glucose and electrolyte balance?

31. Describe specific assessments needed before and during the use of ritodrine or terbutaline.

32. What are the baseline laboratory studies needed before the initiation of ritodrine therapy?

33. Describe the potential effects of ritodrine on the neonate.

34. For what clinical condition is clomiphene citrate used?

35. Identify the preliminary screening needed before initiation of clomiphene citrate therapy.

36. What safety precautions are needed in the event that visual disturbances occur with the use of clomiphene citrate?
37. At what specific time during the menstrual cycle can ovulation be anticipated with the use of clomiphene citrate?

38. What is the action of magnesium sulfate on the central nervous system?
39. What is the normal range of blood levels of magnesium sulfate when it is used as an anticonvulsant?
40. Prepare a list of assessments that should be implemented during the administration of magnesium sulfate to detect toxicity.

27. Oxytocin can alter fluid balance by stimulating antidiuretic hormone, causing the body to accumulate water. Signs and symptoms include drowsiness, listlessness, headache, confusion, oliguria, edema, and in extreme cases, seizures.
28. Uterine stimulants increase uterine activity. Uterine relaxants are used to delay or prevent labor and delivery in selected patients.

29. Adrenergic or sympathetic control
Beta$_1$: Increase rate and force of heart contractions.
Beta$_2$: Relaxation of smooth muscles in bronchi, uterus, gastrointestinal tract, and peripheral vascular area. Monitor for tachycardia and hypotension.
30. May cause hyperglycemia because of stimulation of the sympathetic system, resulting in an increase in glycogenolysis. Continuous, long-term infusions of ritodrine or terbutaline may also cause hypokalemia. Monitor serum electrolytes periodically.
31. Obtain baseline vital signs and weight. Monitor maternal and fetal heart rates. Perform baseline mental status assessment (e.g., alertness, orientation, anxiety level, muscle strength, tremors). Monitor diabetic patients for hyperglycemia.
32. Serum glucose, chloride, sodium, potassium, hematocrit, and carbon dioxide before initiation of therapy.
33. Neonatal adverse effects include hyperglycemia followed by hypoglycemia, hypotension, hypocalcemia and paralytic ileus.
34. It is used to induce ovulation in women who are not ovulating because of reduced circulating estrogen levels.
35. A complete physical exam must rule out other pathologic causes for lack of ovulation.

36. See a physician for an eye exam. Avoid tasks requiring visual acuity (e.g., driving or operating power machinery). Visual disturbances usually subside in a few days to weeks following discontinuation of the medication.
37. Usually 6 to 10 days after the last dose of medication.

38. It depresses the central nervous system (CNS) and blocks peripheral nerve transmission, causing muscle relaxation.
39. 4 to 8 mEq/L

Copyright © 2001 by Mosby, Inc. All rights reserved.

41. Explain the rationale for monitoring urine output during magnesium sulfate therapy.

42. What methods are used to assess deep tendon reflexes and what specific findings would require notification of the physician?
43. Identify treatment for magnesium sulfate toxicity.
44. Describe specific procedures and precautions needed during the intravenous administration of magnesium sulfate.
45. What nursing assessments are needed to monitor infants born to mothers receiving magnesium sulfate?
46. What emergency supplies should be available in the immediate vicinity during magnesium sulfate therapy?
47. What are the action and purpose of administration of Rh$_o$(D) immune globulin?

48. Identify the specific dosage, administration precautions, and proper timing of the administration of Rh$_o$(D) immune globulin.

49. State the appropriate treatment of fever, arthralgia, and generalized aches and pains that can be anticipated following Rh$_o$(D) immune globulin administration.
50. What is the purpose of erythromycin ophthalmic ointment?
51. Describe the specific procedures used to instill erythromycin ophthalmic ointment.

52. What is the causative organism of ophthalmia neonatorum?
53. Explain the rationale for administering phytonadione to the neonate.
54. What is the preferred site for intramuscular administration of Vitamin K to a neonate?

55. Review the anatomical structures associated with the administration of intramuscular medications in an infant.
56. What side effects to report are associated with phytonadione therapy?

40. Deep tendon reflexes: Patellar reflex qh (IV), or before every dose IM. Hourly urine output: Report output of less than 30 ml/hour or less than 100 ml/4 hours. Vital signs: Take q 15 to 30 minutes. Respirations must be at least 16/minute before further doses are administered. If blood pressure drops, do not administer another dose. Fetal distress: do not administer. Mental status: check orientation and alertness before initiating therapy.
41. With reduced urine output, toxicity is more likely to occur.

42. See text on Deep Tendon Reflex, p. 489.
43. Administer calcium gluconate 10%. Stop magnesium infusion.

44. Use an infusion pump. Periodic neurologic exam, I & O, fetal assessment, vital signs.

45. Monitor for hyporeflexia and respiratory depression. May also be hypotensive.

46. Calcium gluconate 10% solution ready for IV administration. Ambu bag, in case of respiratory depression. Discontinue the IV infusion.
47. It is used to prevent Rh immunization of the Rh– patient exposed to Rh+ blood as a result of a transfusion accident, during termination of pregnancy, or as a result of a delivery of an Rh+ infant. Action: Prevents Rh hemolytic disease in subsequent delivery.
48. See drug monograph, p. 490.

49. Use acetaminophen, not aspirin or other anti-inflammatory agents.
50. Used prophylactically to prevent ophthalmia neonatorum caused by *Neisseria gonorrhoeae* or *Chlamydia trachomatis*
51. See Therapeutic Outcome, textbook p. 491.

52. *Neisseria gonorrhoeae* or *Chlamydia trachomatis*.

53. Newborns are often deficient in bacteria to produce Vitamin K. They are also deficient in clotting factors and are more susceptible to hemorrhagic disease.
54. Lateral aspect of the thigh.

55. See Parenteral Medications and Administration of Medication by the Intramuscular Route (pp. 119-125).
56. Bruising, hemorrhage, petechiae, bleeding from any site or orifice.

Copyright © 2001 by Mosby, Inc. All rights reserved.

Practice Quiz

Drugs Used in Obstetrics

ESSAY

1. When magnesium sulfate is administered, what emergency supplies should be available in the immediate vicinity?
2. Why is $Rh_o(D)$ immune globulin (RhoGAM) administered to a mother after delivery?
3. List assessments and nursing interventions needed for an individual who develops pregnancy-induced hypertension (PIH).
4. How often should the deep tendon reflexes be monitored in a patient receiving magnesium sulfate?
5. What is the antidote for magnesium sulfate toxicity?
6. Explain the procedure used following delivery to prevent ophthalmia neonatorum.
7. Why is phytonadione (AquaMEPHYTON) administered to a newborn?
8. What premedication assessments should be done prior to oxytocin administration?

END-OF-CHAPTER MATH REVIEW

1. Ordered: Methylergonovine maleate (Methergine) 0.2 mg IM immediately after delivery of the placenta.
   On hand: Check the drug monograph in the textbook to determine the availability of the drug.
   Give: _____ ml.
2. Ordered: Magnesium sulfate 1 g/hr by continuous infusion
   On hand: Magnesium sulfate 4 g added to 250 ml 5% D/W
   Set the infusion pump at: _____ ml/hr

CRITICAL THINKING QUESTIONS

1. After delivery of a newborn, an Rh– mother asks why she must receive RhoGAM. Give an explanation of the rationale that a lay person would understand.
2. Why is it necessary to prehydrate the mother before administration of terbutaline IV?
3. During administration of terbutaline IV, the woman's pulse elevates to 150 beats per minute and the fetal heart rate is 200 beats/minute. What actions would you take?

Copyright © 2001 by Mosby, Inc. All rights reserved.

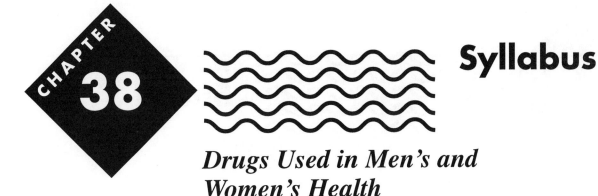

CHAPTER 38

Drugs Used in Men's and Women's Health

Syllabus

CHAPTER CONTENTS

CHAPTER OBJECTIVES

1. Identify common organisms known to cause leukorrhea.
2. Cite the generic and brand names of products used to treat *Candida albicans, Trichomonas vaginalis,* and *Gardnerella vaginalis.*
3. Review specific techniques for administering vaginal medications.
4. Develop a plan for teaching self-care to women and men with sexually transmitted diseases. Include personal hygiene measures, medication administration, methods of pain relief, and prevention of spread of infection or reinfection.
5. Discuss specific interviewing techniques that can be used to obtain a patient's history of sexual activity.
6. Compare the active ingredients in the two types of oral contraceptive agents.
7. Differentiate between the actions and the benefits of the combination pill and the minipill.
8. Describe the major adverse effects of and contraindications to the use of oral contraceptive agents.
9. Develop specific patient education plans to be used to teach a patient to initiate oral contraceptive therapy with the combination pill and the minipill.

10. Describe pharmacological treatments of benign prostatic hyperplasia.
11. Describe the pharmacologic treatment of erectile dysfunction.

KEY WORDS

leukorrhea
dysmenorrhea
sexually transmitted diseases

ASSIGNMENTS

Read textbook pp. 492-506.
Study Key Words associated with chapter content.
Study Review Sheet for Chapter 38.
Complete End-of-Chapter Math Review and Critical
    Thinking Questions.
Complete the Collaborative Activity as assigned by
    instructor.
Complete Chapter 38 Practice Quiz.
Complete Chapter 38 Exam.

COLLABORATIVE ACTIVITY

Complete the following as preparation for in-class discussion and group work that may be assigned by the instructor.

Develop a health teaching plan for a woman with a vaginal infection.

Copyright © 2001 by Mosby, Inc.   All rights reserved.

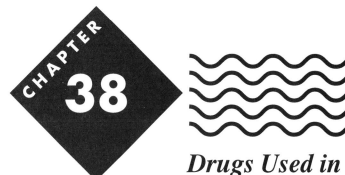

Review Sheet

Drugs Used in Men's and Women's Health

The QUESTION column and the ANSWER column have been offset so that you can cover the answers while reading the questions, allowing you to assess your knowledge.

Question	**Answer**
1. Define *leukorrhea*.	
2. What types of infection are known to develop in the mouth, gastrointestinal tract, or vagina with the use of broad spectrum antibiotics?	1. Leukorrhea is an abnormal, usually whitish vaginal discharge.
3. List the diseases collectively known as sexually transmitted diseases (STD).	2. *C. albicans* and others listed in Table 38-2.
4. Identify the components of a female and/or male reproductive history.	3. See Table 38-3, p. 496.
5. What history of drug use would be of significance in a medication history and should be reported to the physician?	4. See textbook, pp. 493-495.
6. List laboratory studies used to detect infection in the male or female reproductive system.	5. Steroids, antibiotics, illegal drugs, allergies, and previous drug treatment of the same condition.
7. Identify basic hygiene measures that should be taught to men and women.	6. Gram stains and cultures from anus, vagina, throat, and urethra. VDRL and rapid/plasma reagin (RPR), fluorescent treponema antibody absorption, tissue cultures for HSV-2, HIV testing, as appropriate tests for STDs.
8. Explain in detail the proper method of applying vaginal medications topically or intravaginally and discuss medication regimens used for both partners in a sexual relationship.	7. See textbook, pp. 496-497.
9. How is a psychosocial assessment that focuses on obtaining data related to sexually transmitted diseases completed?	8. Patient Education and Health Promotion, Medications. Textbook, p. 497.
10. Compare the active ingredients of combination and progestin-only oral contraceptive agents.	9. See textbook, p. 494.
11. Differentiate between the actions and the benefits of the combination pill and the minipill oral contraceptives.	10. See textbook, p. 497.

Copyright © 2001 by Mosby, Inc.   All rights reserved.

12. Describe the major adverse effects of and contraindications for the use of oral contraceptives.

13. Develop a specific education plan for teaching patients about oral contraceptives.

14. What medications, when combined with oral contraceptive therapy, require the use of an alternate form of contraceptive therapy?

15. Differentiate between the symptoms of obstructive and irritative benign prostatic hypertrophy.

16. Compare the actions of alpha$_1$ adrenergic blocking agents and antiandrogen agents on the prostatic gland.

17. What is androgenetic alopecia?

18. What premedication assessments should be made prior to administering alpha$_1$ adrenergic blocking agents and antiandrogen agents?

19. Define erectile dysfunction and differentiate between vascular, neurologic, and psychologic causative factors.

20. Why is it important to check for a history of cardiovascular disease before initiating sildenafil (Viagra) therapy?

21. What is the time of onset and duration of action of sildenafil?

11. The combination pill prevents conception by inhibiting ovulation, by making the cervical mucus thick and inhibiting sperm migration, and by impairing implantation of the fertilized ovum. The minipill prevents conception through progestin activity on cervical mucus, uterine and fallopian transport, and implantation.

12. Diseases that may be aggravated by oral contraceptive therapy include hypertension, gallbladder disease, diabetes mellitus, severe varicose veins, seizure disorders, oligomenorrhea or amenorrhea, and rheumatic heart disease. Side effects common with oral contraceptive therapy are nausea, headache, weight gain, spotting, depression, fatigue, chloasma, yeast infections, vaginal itching or discharge, and changes in libido.

13. See textbook, Oral Contraceptive Therapy: Administration, p. 501.

14. Ampicillin, isoniazid, rifampin, phenytoin, primidone, carbamazepine, phenobarbital.

15. See Table 38-5, p. 500.

16. Alpha$_1$ adrenergic blocking agents relax the smooth muscles of the bladder and prostate, whereas antiandrogen agents block androgens at the prostate cellular level and cause the prostate gland to shrink.

17. Male pattern baldness. Elevated dihydrotestosterone (DHT) induces androgenetic alopecia.

18. See textbook, pp. 503-504.

19. See textbook, p. 504.

20. Sildenafil can cause fatal interactions with nitroglycerin or isosorbide. Always check with a physician if a patient has any history of cardiovascular disease before initiating therapy.

21. Take one-half to four hours before sexual activity; erectile function lasts for an hour or more but is highly variable and dependent on a number of factors.

Copyright © 2001 by Mosby, Inc.   All rights reserved.

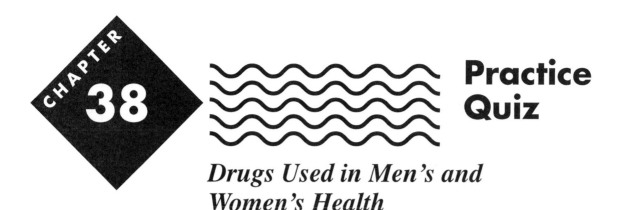

CHAPTER 38

Drugs Used in Men's and Women's Health

Practice Quiz

COMPLETION

Complete the following statements.

The combination pill contains 1. _____ and _____ hormones. These hormones are taken for 2. _____ days per month.

The progestin-only oral contraceptive is taken 3. _____ day of the month. This type of oral contraceptive is called the 4. _____ .

List five common side effects associated with contraceptive therapy:

5. _____

6. _____

7. _____

8. _____

9. _____

ESSAY

10. Describe personal hygiene measures that should be taught to males and females being treated for sexually transmitted infectious diseases.
11. What medications are known to decrease or inhibit the effectiveness of oral contraceptive therapy?
12. What two classifications of drugs are used in the treatment of benign prostatic hyperplasia?
13. How does finasteride effect the results of a serum PSA level?
14. What premedication assessments should be performed before beginning sildenafil therapy?

END-OF-CHAPTER MATH REVIEW

1. Ordered: Acyclovir (Zovirax) 200 mg po q 4 h while awake for a total of five capsules per day.
   The total daily dose would be _____mg.
   A prescription that is to last for two weeks until the patient is seen in the clinic again would need to have a total of _____ capsules.
2. Ordered: Doxycycline (Doryx) 100 mg q 12 h po for the first day; followed by 100 mg/day po for a total of 10 days.
   When the prescription comes from the pharmacy, how many capsules should be in the bottle (the product is available in 100 mg capsules)?
   _____ capsules

CRITICAL THINKING QUESTIONS

1. A.J. is being started on a combination oral contraceptive. You are to give her the initial health teaching regarding the prescription. What would you explain?
2. S.W. comes to the clinic for an annual physical and renewal of her oral contraceptives. She tests positive for Chlamydia and becomes very upset when informed of this. How would you address this situation?
3. A neighbor tells you he is obtaining Viagra through the "black market." What should you do in view of your knowledge of this drug and its action and potential interactions?

Copyright © 2001 by Mosby, Inc.   All rights reserved.

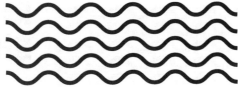 **Syllabus**

Drugs Used to Treat Disorders of the Urinary System

CHAPTER CONTENTS

CHAPTER OBJECTIVES

1. Explain the major actions and effects of drugs used to treat disorders of the urinary tract.
2. Identify baseline data the nurse should collect on a continuous basis for comparison and evaluation of drug effectiveness.
3. Identify important nursing assessments and interventions associated with drug therapy and treatment of diseases of the urinary system.
4. Identify essential components involved in planning patient education that will enhance compliance with the treatment regimen.
5. Analyze Table 39-1 and identify specific portions of a urinalysis report that would indicate proteinuria, dehydration, infection, or renal disease.
6. Prepare a chart of antimicrobial agents used to treat urinary tract infections. Give the drug names, the organisms treated, and special considerations (e.g., need for acidic urine, changes in urine color, effect on urine tests).
7. Develop a health teaching plan for an individual who has repeated urinary tract infections.

KEY WORDS

pyelonephritis
cystitis
prostatitis
urethritis

antispasmodic agent
acidification
neurogenic bladder

ASSIGNMENTS

Read textbook pp. 507-516.
Study Key Words associated with chapter content.
Study Review Sheet for Chapter 39.
Complete End-of-Chapter Math Review and Critical Thinking Questions.
Complete the Collaborative Activity as assigned by instructor.
Complete Chapter 39 Practice Quiz.
Complete Chapter 39 Exam.

COLLABORATIVE ACTIVITY

Complete the following as preparation for in-class discussion and group work that may be assigned by the instructor.

Compare the premedication assessments needed for fosfomycins, quinolones, and bladder-active agents.

Copyright © 2001 by Mosby, Inc.   All rights reserved.

CHAPTER 39

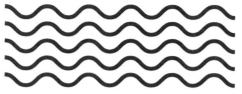

Review Sheet

Drugs Used to Treat Disorders of the Urinary System

The QUESTION column and the ANSWER column have been offset so that you can cover the answers while reading the questions, allowing you to assess your knowledge.

Question	Answer
1. Differentiate between pyelonephritis, cystitis, prostatitis, and urethritis.	
2. Why is the use of strict aseptic technique needed with indwelling catheters?	1. Pyelonephritis is kidney infection, cystitis is bladder infection, prostatitis is prostate gland infection, and urethritis is infection of the urethra.
3. In the elderly, what is a common sign of a UTI?	2. Prevent urinary tract infections (UTIs).
4. Study Table 39-1 to identify details found on a routine urinalysis report.	3. Confusion
5. What measures should be taught to prevent UTIs?	4. See Table 39-1, textbook p. 509.
6. Name a urinary analgesic and describe its action.	5. Personal hygiene measures—wiping front to back in female; keeping perineal area clean; avoiding nylon underwear and constrictive clothing in perineal area; avoiding scented bubble bath products and colored toilet paper; washing the perineal area immediately before and after intercourse; and urinating after intercourse.
7. What changes in urine color can often occur following the administration of phenazopyridine?	6. Phenazopyridine hydrochloride (Pyridium) acts as a local anesthetic on the mucosa of the ureters and bladder, reducing spasm.
8. Should a urine specimen for bacterial culture and sensitivity be collected before or after starting antimicrobial therapy?	7. Reddish-orange urine. Inform the patient not to be alarmed.
9. What health teaching should be completed when a patient has a urinary tract infection?	8. Before giving the first dose of an antimicrobial agent.
10. Why must the urine be acidic during the administration of methenamine mandelate (Mandelamine)?	9. Force fluids, 2000 ml or more per day. Continue medication for the entire course of treatment, even if symptoms have subsided fairly rapidly. Return for urine culture when scheduled. Have patient report perineal itching, vaginal discharge, or breakdown of tissue. Teach the patient ways to prevent future infections.

 Copyright © 2001 by Mosby, Inc. All rights reserved.

11. Urine pH should be maintained below what value for optimal results from methenamine mandelate therapy?

12. Why are some urinary antimicrobial agents prescribed to be taken after the urine culture is sterile?
13. What color change in the urine may occur with nitrofurantoin therapy?
14. Which urinary antimicrobial agent is more likely to cause photosensitivity?
15. Name two medicines that may be used in nonobstructive urinary retention (e.g., postoperatively, during postpartum period).
16. What drug should be readily available for treatment of serious adverse effects of bethanechol?
17. Identify the components of an assessment of the urinary tract.
18. What are the desired therapeutic outcomes of therapy with quinoline type drugs?
19. What drug class is newly approved for one-time treatment of urinary tract infections?
20. What types of urinary tract organisms can be successfully treated with quinolone antibiotics or nitrofurantoin?
21. What type of anemia precludes the use of quinolone antibiotics?
22. How is urinary tract acidification accomplished?
23. What drugs cause alkalinization of the urine?

10. In order for methenamine mandelate (Mandelamine) to be effective it must be converted to formaldehyde to suppress the growth of bacteria. The urine has to be acidic for this reaction to occur. Therefore, the patient may have vitamin C prescribed simultaneously for this purpose.
11. When the pH is above 5.5, methenamine is less likely to be converted to formaldehyde.

12. To prevent recurrent urinary tract infection.

13. Urine may become tinted yellow to rust-brown.

14. Nalidixic acid (NegGram).

15. Bethanechol chloride (Urecholine) and neostigmine (Prostigmin)
16. Atropine sulfate

17. See textbook, p. 508.

18. Resolution of the urinary tract infection

19. Fosfomycin antibiotics (Fosfomycin, Monurol)

20. See textbook, pp. 511-512.

21. Glucose-6-phosphate dehydrogenase deficiency.
22. Vitamin C
23. Acetazolamide and sodium bicarbonate

Copyright © 2001 by Mosby, Inc. All rights reserved.

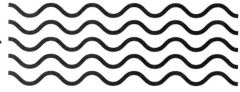

Practice Quiz

Drugs Used to Treat Disorders of the Urinary System

ESSAY

1. When an individual complains of urinary tract symptoms (e.g., urinary frequency, pain, or retention) he or she should have what nursing interventions?
2. When phenazopyridine hydrochloride is administered, the patient should be counseled that the urine will be what color?
3. How can the urine be acidified?
4. What class of drugs should not be administered to patients with a known glucose-6-phosphate dehydrogenase deficiency?

COMPLETION

Complete the following statements.

5. In the presence of acidic urine, methenamine mandelate (Mandelamine) forms _____.
6. Nitrofurantoin is an effective antibiotic for systemic infections. (True or False)
7. The urine color that may occur with Macrodantin therapy is _____.
8. Urecholine and Prostigmine are used to treat what urinary disorder _____?
9. The class of antibiotic used for single dose treatment of a urinary tract infection is _____.
10. In order for methenamine mandelate (Mandelamine) to be active the urine must be _____.
11. The medication used to acidify urine is _____.
12. Persons taking nitrofurantoin should be told the color of the urine may be _____.
13. Drugs used to treat nonobstructive urinary tract retention include _____.

END-OF-CHAPTER MATH REVIEW

1. Ordered: Bethanechol chloride (Urecholine) 2.5 mg sc stat
   On hand: Bethanechol chloride 5 mg/ml.
   Give: _____ ml
2. Ordered: Methenamine mandelate (Mandelamine) 750 mg po
   On hand: Methenamine mandelate 0.5 g/5 ml suspension
   Give: _____ ml

CRITICAL THINKING QUESTION

Situation: M.C., age 64, a resident of Longmeadow Nursing Home, has developed her third urinary tract infection (UTI) in the past four months.

1. What assessments should be made? Discuss appropriate nursing actions during the treatment of the current urinary tract infection and measures to prevent another episode.

Copyright © 2001 by Mosby, Inc.   All rights reserved.

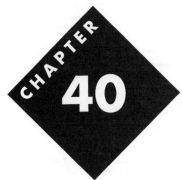

CHAPTER 40

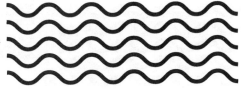

Syllabus

Drugs Used to Treat Glaucoma and Other Eye Disorders

CHAPTER CONTENTS

CHAPTER OBJECTIVES

1. Describe the normal flow of aqueous humor in the eye.
2. Identify the changes in normal flow of aqueous humor caused by open-angle and closed-angle glaucoma.
3. Explain baseline data that should be gathered when an eye disorder exists.
4. Review the correct procedure for instilling eye drops or eye ointments.
5. Develop teaching plans for a person with an eye infection and one receiving glaucoma medication.

KEY WORDS

cornea	near point
sclera	zonular fibers
iris	cycloplegia
sphincter muscle	lacrimal canaliculi
miosis	intraocular pressure
dilator muscle	closed-angle glaucoma
mydriasis	open-angle glaucoma
lens	

ASSIGNMENTS

Read textbook pp. 517-533.
Study Key Words associated with chapter content.
Study Review Sheet for Chapter 40.
Complete End-of-Chapter Math Review and Critical
    Thinking Questions.
Complete Collaborative Activities as assigned by
    instructor.
Complete Chapter 40 Practice Quiz.
Complete Chapter 40 Exam.

COLLABORATIVE ACTIVITIES

Complete the following as preparation for in-class discussion and group work that may be assigned by the instructor.

B.G. is a 55-year-old male who was found to have an elevated intraocular pressure in both eyes on routine examination. Further examination revealed cupping of the optic discs and a nerve fiber bundle defect consistent with glaucoma. Gonioscopy indicated that the anterior chamber angles were open in both eyes. Upon questioning, B.G. related a family history of glaucoma. B.G.'s diagnosis is primary open-angle glaucoma of genetic origin. A prescription order was written to start treatment:
    Timolol 0.25% 1 drop in each eye twice daily

1. What is the action of the medicine prescribed?
2. Explain the procedure the nurse would use to teach the patient to administer this medication.
3. What additional patient education should be performed?

Copyright © 2001 by Mosby, Inc.   All rights reserved.

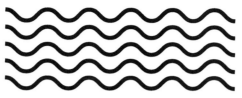

Review Sheet

Drugs Used to Treat Glaucoma and Other Eye Disorders

The QUESTION column and the ANSWER column have been offset so that you can cover the answers while reading the questions, allowing you to assess your knowledge.

Question	Answer
1. Identify the major structures of the eye (e.g., cornea, pupil, iris, Canal of Schlemm).	
2. Define *accommodation, cycloplegia, exophthalmos, glaucoma, miosis, mydriasis,* and *refraction.*	1. Refer to textbook for a review of the basic structure and function of the eye. In particular, examine the location of the Canal of Schlemm, Fig. 40-3. Note that dilation of the iris could result in a blockage of the Canal of Schlemm.
	2. Accommodation: The adjustment of the lens for near or far vision. Cycloplegia: Paralysis of the ciliary muscles. Exophthalmos: Bulging of the eyeball or abnormal protrusion of the eyeball. Glaucoma: An eye disorder characterized by an increase in the intraocular pressure. Miosis: Contraction of the iris sphincter muscle causing narrowing of the pupil of the eye. Mydriasis: Contraction of the dilator muscle and relaxation of the sphincter muscle causing dilation of the pupil of the eye. Refraction: An eye exam that determines whether an individual needs to wear glasses.
3. Explain the normal drainage system of the eye.	3. Aqueous humor flows between the lens and the iris into the anterior chamber of the eye. It drains through channels located near the junction of the cornea and the sclera through meshwork into the Canal of Schlemm and then into the venous system of the eye.
4. Identify the normal intraocular pressure reading when taken with a tonometer.	4. 10 to 21 mmHg
5. Compare the mechanisms of action of drugs used to lower intraocular pressure.	5. Osmotic agents: elevate osmotic pressure of the plasma, causing fluid from the extravascular spaces to be drawn into the blood thereby reducing intraocular pressure (IOP).
6. Describe the actions of drugs known as mydriatic agents and miotic agents.	Carbonic anhydrase inhibitors: inhibit the enzyme carbonic anhydrase which results in a decrease of aqueous humor production thereby lowering IOP.
	Cholinergic agents: produce contraction of the iris (miosis) and ciliary body musculature (accommodation), thereby permitting outflow of

Copyright © 2001 by Mosby, Inc.   All rights reserved.

aqueous humor by widening the filtration angle, thus decreasing IOP.

Cholinesterase inhibitors: prevent destruction of acetylcholine, the cholinergic neurotransmitter within the eye. This results in increased cholinergic activity because of miosis the IOP is reduced.

Adrenergic agents: have several uses in ophthalmology. These agents cause pupil dilation, increased outflow of aqueous humor, vasoconstriction, relaxation of ciliary muscle, and decreased formation of aqueous humor.

Beta-adrenergic blocking agents are thought to reduce production of aqueous humor.

Prostaglandin agonists increase outflow of aqueous humor.

7. What should the nurse look for when performing an assessment of the pupil?

8. Cholinergic agents cause the pupil to _____.

9. List common side effects of cholinergic agents.

10. Explain how the systemic effects of cholinergic agents can be minimized.

11. Cholinesterase inhibitors block the destruction of what neurotransmitter, causing prolonged cholinergic activity and resulting in miosis and decreased intraocular pressure?

12. An overdose of a cholinesterase inhibitor will cause what symptoms?

13. Adrenergic agents cause pupil _____, and a _____ in formation of _____.

14. Adrenergic blocking agents _____ intraocular pressure.

15. What types of patients should not receive beta-adrenergic blocking agents?

16. What action does an osmotic diuretic have on the IOP?

17. Side effects from osmotic agents that can be anticipated include:

18. Osmotic agents may produce fluid overload or heart failure. Signs and symptoms of this include:

19. Describe the nursing assessments needed during the administration of osmotic agents.

6. Mydriatic agents dilate the pupil and miotic agents constrict the pupil.

7. Pupil size, shape, and accommodation when exposed to light.

8. Constrict; this increases or widens the filtration angle near the Canal of Schlemm, permitting outflow of the aqueous humor.

9. Reduced visual acuity, conjunctival irritation, headache, pain, and discomfort.

10. To reduce systemic absorption from the highly vascular nasal tissues, block the inner canthus of the eye for 1 to 2 minutes immediately after instilling the eye drop(s).

11. Acetylcholine

12. Systemic toxicity manifested by sweating, salivation, vomiting, abdominal cramping, urinary incontinence, diarrhea, bronchospasms, arrhythmias, and bradycardia.

13. Dilation; decrease; aqueous humor

14. Reduce IOP; also may reduce production of aqueous humor.

15. Patients with a respiratory condition (e.g., bronchitis, emphysema, and asthma) because beta blockers may produce severe bronchoconstriction. Use in patients with heart failure should be limited to those persons whose disease is under control because hypotension, bradycardia, and/or heart failure may develop with use of these agents.

16. Osmotic agents reduce the volume of intraocular fluid present.

17. Thirst, nausea, dehydration, electrolyte imbalance (potassium, sodium, and chloride), headache, and circulatory overload.

18. Fluid overload/pulmonary edema, apprehension, cyanosis, diaphoresis, rapid pulse, dyspnea, and moist, gurgling-type respirations. Patients may also develop a productive cough with frothy, pink-tinged sputum.

Copyright © 2001 by Mosby, Inc.   All rights reserved.   **203**

20. Before administering a carbonic anhydrase inhibitor, the nurse should check the patient's chart for _____.

21. The class of drugs that produces both mydriasis and cycloplegia is _____.
22. To what drug classification does latanoprost (Xalatan) belong?
23. When mydriatic agents are administered, what patient reaction to bright lights is seen?
24. What specific medication is used to treat an ophthalmic fungal infection?
25. Antiviral agents may produce what adverse effects?
26. What is the major use of corticosteroid therapy in the eye?
27. What eye complications can occur with the long-term use of corticosteroids?
28. What is the desired action of an antihistamine on eye disorders?

29. Review the procedures and abbreviations used for administering eye medications.
30. The drug sodium fluorescein is used for what purpose?

31. When are artificial tears used?

19. Check urinary output frequently and record the amount accurately. An indwelling catheter is usually inserted, depending on the circumstances. Assess the intravenous site q 15 min, and take vital signs q 15 min, or more frequently, as ordered. Check the rate of infusion at least q 30 minutes.
20. A history of allergy to sulfonamides

21. Anticholinergic agents

22. Prostaglandin agonist

23. Squinting because of excessive dilation; reduced visual acuity
24. Natamycin (Natacyn)
25. Sensitivity to bright lights, visual haze, lacrimation, redness, and burning
26. For allergic reactions of the eye and other acute, noninfectious inflammatory conditions of the eye
27. Increased IOP, glaucoma, and cataracts.
   Do not use with bacterial fungal or viral infections of the eye because corticosteroids decrease defense mechanisms and reduce resistance to pathologic organisms.
28. Antihistamines relieve signs and symptoms and prevent itching associated with allergic conjunctivitis.
29. os = left eye
   od = right eye
   ou = both eyes (See textbook p. 147.)
30. Fitting hard contact lenses and as diagnostic aid to identify foreign bodies in the eye or corneal abrasions.
31. Artificial tear solutions are products made to mimic natural secretions of the eye. They provide lubrication for dry eyes and for artificial eyes. They are also used to prevent drying when a person has lost the blink reflex such as during surgery or when comatose.

Copyright © 2001 by Mosby, Inc. All rights reserved.

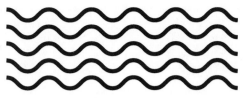

Practice Quiz

Drugs Used to Treat Glaucoma and Other Eye Disorders

COMPLETION

Complete the following statements.

The abbreviation 1. _____ means left eye, 2. _____ means right eye, and 3. _____ means both eyes.

When administering eye medications, it is important to 4. _____ for 5. _____ minutes immediately after instilling the eye drops to minimize systemic effects.

Cholinesterase inhibitors destroy cholinesterase, an enzyme that destroys the neurotransmitter 6. _____. The prolonged action of the neurotransmitter lowers intraocular pressure and 7. _____ of the pupil.

Adrenergic agents cause 8. _____ of the pupil.

The action of osmotic agents on glaucoma is to 9. _____.

The mechanism of action of carbonic anhydrase inhibitors used to treat glaucoma is 10. _____.

Antiviral agents may cause what side effects (list minimum of 4):
11. _____
_____
_____
_____

Corticosteroids are used in the eye to 12. _____.

When carbonic anhydrase inhibitors are administered, intraocular pressure is reduced by 13._____.

Beta adrenergic blocking agents should not be administered to patients with 14._____.

END-OF-CHAPTER MATH REVIEW

1. Ordered: 1.5 g/kg mannitol 15% solution IV over 30 minutes.
   The patient weighs 156 lbs. What is the weight in kg:____?
   The total g of mannitol to administer is: _____

CRITICAL THINKING QUESTIONS

1. While working in the eye clinic, the nurse observes that several of the patients being treated for glaucoma complain that the medications cause pain and headache and that reading ability is diminished. How would you respond to these statements?
2. Develop a teaching plan for a patient who is to self-administer Betoptic one drop twice daily.

Copyright © 2001 by Mosby, Inc. All rights reserved.

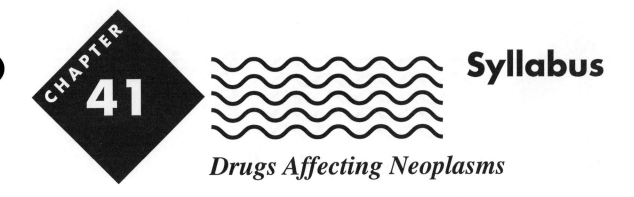

Syllabus

Drugs Affecting Neoplasms

CHAPTER CONTENT

Cancer and the Use of Antineoplastic Agents (p. 535)
Drug Therapy (p. 535)
    Drug Class: Alkylating Agents (p. 546)
    Drug Class: Antibiotics (p. 546)
    Drug Class: Antimetabolites (p. 546)
    Drug Class: Natural Products (p. 546)
    Drug Class: Hormones (p. 548)

CHAPTER OBJECTIVES

1. Cite the goals of chemotherapy.
2. Explain the normal cycle for cell replication and describe the effects of cell cycle-specific and cell cycle-nonspecific drugs within this process.
3. Cite the rationale for giving chemotherapeutic drugs on a precise time schedule.
4. State which types of chemotherapeutic agents are cell-cycle specific and those that are cell-cycle nonspecific.
5. Describe the role of immunomodulators and chemoprotective agents in treating cancer.
6. Study the nursing assessments and interventions needed for persons experiencing adverse effects from chemotherapy.
7. Develop patient education objectives for a patient receiving chemotherapy.

KEY WORDS

cancer
metastases
cell cycle-specific
cell cycle-nonspecific
palliation

combination therapy
immunomodulators
chemoprotective agents
adjuvant therapy
intermittent therapy

ASSIGNMENTS

Read textbook pp. 534-548.
Study Key Words associated with chapter content.
Study Review Sheet for Chapter 41.
Complete End-of-Chapter Math Review and Critical Thinking Questions.
Complete Collaborative Activities as assigned by instructor.
Complete Chapter 41 Practice Quiz.
Complete Chapter 41 Exam.

COLLABORATIVE ACTIVITIES

Complete the following as preparation for in-class discussion and group work that may be assigned by the instructor.

Many times a cancer patient will have an order for administration of a biologic response modifier. Research the following drugs:
1. Epoetin (Epogen, Procrit):
   What is the action of epoetin on blood cells?
   Why is epoetin also used in end-stage renal disease?
   What premedication assessments should be made prior to epoetin administration? What side effects may occur after the drug is administered?
2. Filgrastim (Neupogen)
   What is the action of filgrastim on blood cells?
   What storage parameters are suggested for this drug?
3. Leucovorin calcium (Wellcovorin)
   What is a "leucovorin rescue"? What is the purpose of a leucovorin rescue and what nursing responsibilities are associated with its administration?
4. Mesna (Mesnex)
   What is the action of this drug? Why is it administered to patients receiving ifosfamide?

Copyright © 2001 by Mosby, Inc.   All rights reserved.

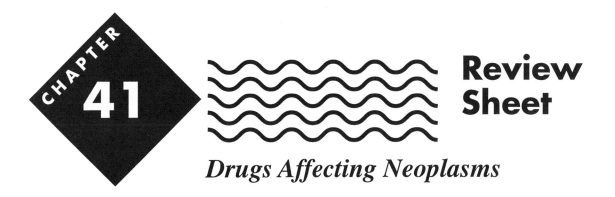

Review Sheet

Drugs Affecting Neoplasms

The QUESTION column and the ANSWER column have been offset so that you can cover the answers while reading the questions, allowing you to assess your knowledge.

Question	Answer
1. What are the phases of the cell cycle?	1. See textbook, p. 535.
2. State baseline assessments needed during the initiation of cancer therapy.	2. The type of cancer being treated, the emotional status of the patient, the understanding the patient has of the diagnosis, the patient's usual methods of coping, the patient's degree of pain, usual eating pattern, and elimination pattern.
3. Cite the goals of chemotherapy and specific factors affecting the patient dosage, drug identification, drug preparation, and drug administration.	3. Control of growth of the cancer cells is the primary goal of treatment. See other goals, textbook p. 535. Since many of the cancer drugs have similar spellings, it is imperative to check the drug name closely. Cancer drugs are given in a variety of forms: orally, intravenously, by bolus, and so forth. Therefore, the physician's order must be checked carefully. Many cancer drugs require reconstitution— follow directions precisely. When drugs are given IV, check the IV site carefully for extravasation. During oral administration, maintain an accurate record of the medication on the flow sheet and record any side effects experienced.
4. State the nursing interventions needed for persons experiencing adverse effects from chemotherapy.	4. See textbook for adverse effects associated with chemotherapy. Monitor for nausea and vomiting, hydration, positioning, changes in bowel patterns, stomatitis, alopecia, neurotoxicity, musculoskeletal complaints, bone marrow depression, infection, thrombocytopenia, and activity intolerance.
5. State the five classes of antineoplastic agents.	5. Alkylating agents, antibiotics, antimetabolites, natural products, and hormones
6. Define cell-cycle specific and cell-cycle nonspecific antineoplastic agents.	6. The action of cell-cycle specific antineoplastic agents occurs in a specific phase of the cell's growth. Cell-cycle nonspecific antineoplastic are active throughout the cell cycle.
7. When is chemotherapy most effective?	7. When cells of the tumor are small in number and rapidly dividing
8. Why is it difficult to kill tumor cells in the G_o phase?	

Copyright © 2001 by Mosby, Inc. All rights reserved.

9. What criteria are used to choose the type of chemotherapy to be administered?

10. Examine Table 41-2, Immunomodulators, and study the action of agents listed. Which agent stimulates production of RBCs?
    Which agent is known as a human granulocyte stimulating factor? Which agent is known as a granulocyte macrophage colony stimulating factor (GM-CSF)?

11. What is/are the action(s) of trastuzumab (Herceptin)?

12. Discuss the three chemoprotective agents amifostine, dexrazoxane, and mesna. What are they primarily used for?

13. List questions that may be asked when taking a health history of the risk factors the individual has for development of cancer.

14. What are the common side effects to expect/report associated with chemotherapy?

15. Why is it sometimes advisable to discuss birth control and reproductive counseling prior to initiation of chemotherapy?

16. What type of oral hygiene measures should be instituted when chemotherapy is administered?

17. What are common signs and symptoms of bleeding the nurse should assess for especially when platelet counts are decreased?

18. What is meant by "neutropenic precautions"?

19. When several courses of intravenously administered chemotherapy are planned, the antineoplastic agents are frequently administered via

    _____.

20. What three types of emesis are associated with antineoplastic therapy?

8. Many chemotherapeutic agents kill cells when in the replication phase. Cells in the resting phase of the cell cycle are not dividing and therefore not susceptible to destruction by chemotherapeutic agents.

9. Type of tumor cells, the rate of growth and size of the tumor.

10. Examine Table 41-2, Immunomodulators. p. 542. Epoietin alpha (Procrit), filgrastim (Neupogen), sargramostim (Leukine)

11. Used in treatment of breast cancer with HER-2 positive tumors. See Table 41-2 for more details.

12. Examine Table 41-3 for detailed discussion.

13. See textbook p. 541.

14. It depends on the type of chemotherapy drug administered. Generally, myelosuppression, anemia, bleeding, stomatitis, diarrhea or constipation, alopecia, anorexia, nausea and vomiting are common symptoms. See a medical-surgical textbook for specific interventions for each of these side effects. Also read implementation and health promotion, pp. 543-546.

15. Reproductive abilities may be affected and agents may pass through the placental barrier; thus being potentially harmful to a fetus.

16. See textbook, pp. 393-394. (See also Chapter 29.)

17. Epistaxis, hematuria, bruises, petechiae, dark, tarry stools, "coffee ground emesis," blurred vision, excessive menstrual flow, hemoglobin, hematocrit.

18. Neutropenic precautions are designed to minimize the individual's exposure to microorganisms. Hand washing, avoiding exposure to individuals with infection, no fresh flowers or fruits and vegetables; no freestanding water (e.g., plants, flowers, humidifiers, denture cups). Avoid pets and persons receiving immunizations.

19. Implantable vascular access devices.

21. Identify whether the following agents are cell-cycle specific or cell-cycle nonspecific: alkylating agents, antimetabolites, natural products, antineoplastic antibiotics. What is the action of hormones?

20. Acute, delayed, and anticipatory emesis (see also Chapter 31).

21. Alkylating agents: cell-cycle nonspecific.
Antimetabolites: Many are cell-cycle specific S phase.
Natural products: Cell-cycle specific
Antineoplastic antibiotics act through various mechanisms to prevent replication as well as RNA synthesis. See drug class for discussion of specific antibiotic agents that are cell cycle specific and cell-cycle nonspecific.
Hormones: Alter the hormone environment of the cell.

 Copyright © 2001 by Mosby, Inc.   All rights reserved.

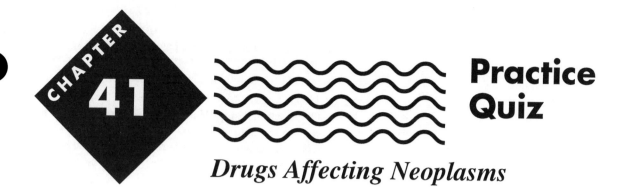

CHAPTER 41

Practice Quiz

Drugs Affecting Neoplasms

COMPLETION

Complete the following statements.

1. R.S. has breast cancer and is receiving chemotherapy with cyclophosphamide, Adriamycin, and fluorouracil. Her latest laboratory report shows:

Patient Report	*Normal Range*
WBC: 3,000	5,000 to 10,000/mm^3
Hgb: 9.5	12 to 16 g/dl
Platelets: 100,000	150,000/mm^3 to 400,000/mm^3
RBC: 4.5	4.0 to 5.0 million/mm^3

   Use available resources to identify significance of this data and then develop nursing diagnosis statements to support your conclusions.

2. List nursing interventions appropriate for neutropenia.

3. Alkylating agents are cell-cycle _____.
4. Antimetabolites are cell-cycle _____.
5. Natural products are cell-cycle _____.
6. The primary therapeutic outcome desired of chemotherapy is _____.
7. When are antiemetics administered in relation to the administration of IV chemotherapy?

8. What data should be collected to assess an individual's hydration status?

9. Describe nursing interventions needed for a neutropenic patient.

10. The patient has 1000 ml lactated Ringer's running at 80 ml/hr. Using a microdrip administration set, at what drip rate per minute should the IV be infused?

Situation: A patient weighing 135 lbs. is to receive 5 mcg/kg/day sc of filgrastim. The drug is available for injection 300 mcg/ml.

11. How many kg does the patient weigh? _____ (Carry conversions to hundredths, round to tenths.)

12. Based on the data given, how many mcg of filgrastim would be administered? Give: _____ mcg.
13. Give _____ ml. of filgrastim.
14. Mesna is used to protect the toxic affects of what drugs on what organ?
15. Oprelvekin (Neumega) stimulates production of

    _____.

16. Trastuzumab (Herceptin) is used in the treatment of

    _____.

END-OF-CHAPTER MATH REVIEW

1. Ordered: Cefazolin 1 g IV q 8 h
    On hand: Cefazolin 1 g diluted in 50 ml 5% dextrose/water
    To administer this medication over a 30-minute period on a pump that is calibrated in ml/hr, at what rate should the pump be set? _____

2. Ordered: PCA morphine sulfate 1 mg/dose with 6 minute lockout/maximum 30 mg/q 4 h
    Discuss how to initiate the PCA setup on this patient and how to set up the initial settings on the PCA pump. Describe when and how to record the amount of morphine sulfate used each shift.

CRITICAL THINKING QUESTIONS

Situation: T.K., age 65, has small cell cancer of the lung with brain and liver metastases. He has had several grand mal seizures in the past month.

   His orders read:
1. Daily weight
2. Assist with ambulation as tolerated
3. Routine vitals
4. Seizure precautions
5. Intake and output
6. Heparin lock the IV
7. Physical therapy consult to assist with plan for self-care at home
8. IV site dressing change q 72 h

Copyright © 2001 by Mosby, Inc. All rights reserved.

9. Medications:
    Folic acid 1 mg po q d
    Multivitamin 1 po q d
    Ensure 1 can tid
    KCl 20 meq po bid
    Normal saline flush 2.5 ml, heparin lock after
    meds.
    Ranitidine 300 mg po q hs
    Ondansetron 32 mg IV, 30 minutes before
    chemotherapy
    Dexamethasone 4 mg IV q 12 h
    Phenytoin 200 mg po qd
    Lorazepam 1 mg po q 12 h

Develop a Kardex for this patient and a Medication
Administration Record that includes the scheduling of
each medication.

For each medication prescribed, state the drug
action and side effects to expect and report.

For IV medications prescribed, state the drug action, rate of administration, dilution for administration,
monitoring required and what type of IV setup would be
required to initiate the intravenous delivery of the medications.

Situation: Mrs. Oakley, age 68, has gastric cancer with
liver metastasis.

She has the following medication orders:

5% Dextrose/0.45% normal saline at 100 ml/hr
Ondansetron 32 mg IV in 50 ml 5% dextrose/water to
run for 15 minutes
Cisplatin 35 mg in 250 ml normal saline to run for 30
minutes
Add mannitol 12.5 g to cisplatin
Leucovorin 20 mg IV push

1. To carry out these orders, what type of an intravenous
    setup would be required?

2. Because you are not "chemo certified" and could not
    start the chemotherapy drugs as a student nurse, what
    nursing responsibilities would you have during the
    execution of these drug orders?

3. What is the action of each medication, side effects to
    expect, and side effects to report?

4. How would you set a pump to deliver the
    ondansetron in 15 minutes? (The pump is calibrated
    in ml/hr.)

5. At what rate would the same type pump be set to
    administer the cisplatin?

Copyright © 2001 by Mosby, Inc.   All rights reserved.

Syllabus

Drugs Used to Treat the Muscular System

CHAPTER CONTENT

Muscle Relaxants and Neuromuscular Blocking Agents
(p. 550)
Drug Therapy (p. 553)
    Drug Class: Centrally Acting Skeletal Muscle
        Relaxants (p. 553)
    Drug Class: Direct-Acting Skeletal Muscle Relaxant
        (p. 554)
    Drug Class: Neuromuscular Blocking Agents (p. 555)

CHAPTER OBJECTIVES

1. Prepare a list of assessment data needed to evaluate a patient with a skeletal muscle disorder.
2. State the nursing assessments needed to monitor therapeutic response and development of side effects to expect and report from skeletal muscle relaxant therapy.
3. Develop a health teaching plan for patients receiving skeletal muscle relaxant therapy.
4. Describe the effect of centrally acting skeletal muscle relaxants on the central nervous system and the safety precautions required during their use.
5. Describe essential components of patient assessment used for patients receiving neuromuscular blocking agents.
6. Locate information on the use of neuromuscular blocking agents in the patient's chart.
7. List the equipment that should be available in the immediate patient care area when neuromuscular blocking agents are to be administered.

8. Describe the physiologic effects of neuromuscular blocking agents.
9. Cite four uses of neuromuscular blocking agents.
10. Identify the effect of neuromuscular blocking agents on consciousness, memory, and the pain threshold.
11. Describe disease conditions that may affect the patient's ability to tolerate the use of neuromuscular blocking agents.
12. List steps required to treat respiratory depression.

KEY WORDS

cerebral palsy
multiple sclerosis
hypercapnia
muscle spasticity
hyperreflexia

clonus
stroke syndrome
neuromuscular blocking
    agents

ASSIGNMENTS

Read textbook pp. 550-556.
Study Key Words associated with chapter content.
Study Review Sheet for Chapter 42.
Complete End-of-Chapter Math Review and Critical
    Thinking Questions.
Complete Chapter 42 Practice Quiz.
Complete Chapter 42 Exam.

Copyright © 2001 by Mosby, Inc.   All rights reserved.

Review Sheet

Drugs Used to Treat the Muscular System

The QUESTION column and the ANSWER column have been offset so that you can cover the answers while reading the questions, allowing you to assess your knowledge.

Question	Answer
1. Describe the nursing assessments needed to evaluate a patient with a skeletal muscle disorder.	
2. What adjustments are usually required during the initial phase when treating an individual with muscle spasms and pain?	1. See textbook, pp. 550-551.
3. What nursing measures can be implemented to alleviate lower back pain?	2. Immobilize and elevate the affected part; range of motion exercises may be prescribed to prevent muscle atrophy and contractures.
4. Immediately following a muscle injury _____ packs will reduce the swelling.	3. Maintain proper body alignment; elevate the head of the bed 15 to 20 degrees and flex the knees slightly. Give prescribed analgesics and muscle relaxants.
5. To decrease swelling following an injury, how should the affected part be treated?	4. Ice packs
6. What two classes of drugs are used to relieve pain and inflammation associated with musculoskeletal disorders?	5. Elevated and immobilized
7. Compare the site of action of centrally acting and direct-acting muscle relaxants.	6. Analgesic agents are used for pain and anti-inflammatory agents are used to reduce the inflammatory response.
8. Both centrally acting and direct-acting skeletal muscle relaxants can produce hepatotoxicity. What are the signs and symptoms of this toxicity?	7. Centrally acting muscle relaxants depress the central nervous system. Their major benefit may be their sedative effects. Direct-acting skeletal muscle relaxants act directly on the skeletal muscle producing generalized, mild weakness of skeletal muscles.
9. What premedication assessments should be made before administering centrally acting skeletal muscle relaxants?	8. Anorexia, nausea, vomiting, jaundice, hepatomegaly, splenomegaly, and abnormal liver function tests (e.g., AST, ALT, LDH).
10. Which class of muscle relaxants can cause photosensitivity?	9. Baseline vital signs, mental status assessment, laboratory studies as ordered (e.g., liver function, complete blood count)
11. What are the primary uses of baclofen?	10. Direct-acting skeletal muscle relaxants
12. Describe the signs of respiratory depression.	11. Baclofen is used to manage muscle spasticity resulting from multiple sclerosis, spinal cord injuries, and other spinal cord diseases.

Copyright © 2001 by Mosby, Inc.   All rights reserved.

13. What laboratory values would be used to confirm hypoxia and hypercapnia?

14. Why are centrally acting muscle relaxants not given to persons with long-term muscle spasticity?
15. What are the uses of dantrolene (Dantrium)?

16. Explain when and why neuromuscular blocking agents are administered.

17. What effect do neuromuscular blocking agents have on consciousness?

18. What nursing assessments should be made when a neuromuscular blocking agent has been administered?
19. Review the drug interactions that enhance therapeutic and toxic effects of neuromuscular blocking agents and identify the three classes of drugs commonly administered that may interact with neuromuscular blocking agents.

20. Where in the patient's chart is administration of a neuromuscular blocking agent recorded?
21. Name common neuromuscular blocking agents by their generic and brand names.
22. What premedication assessments should be done prior to the administration of a neuromuscular blocking agent?
23. Explain the treatment of overdose of neuromuscular blocking agents.

12. Early signs: restlessness, anxiety, decreased mental alertness, headache, increase in heart rate, blood pressure, and respiratory rate. Later signs: heart rate increases, blood pressure decreases, cyanosis, use of accessory chest, abdominal, and neck muscles in respiratory effort, flaring nostrils. Changes in mental status: confusion progressing to coma.
13. Hypercapnia (elevated pCO_2), hypoxemia (decreased pO_2), and decreased oxygen saturation (SaO_2)
14. They would further reduce the functioning of the individual by reducing the overall strength of the remaining active muscle fibers.
15. Control spasticity of chronic disorders (e.g., cerebral palsy, multiple sclerosis, spinal cord injury, stroke syndrome). Dantrolene is also used to treat neuroleptic malignant syndrome.
16. To provide muscle relaxation during anesthesia; to facilitate endotracheal intubation and prevent laryngospasm; to decrease muscular activity in electroshock therapy; to aid in reducing muscle spasms associated with tetanus.
17. No effects. Unless anesthetized, the patient is fully conscious but unable to respond due to neuromuscular blockade.
18. Patent, adequate airway, check lung sounds bilaterally. Residual effects may be apparent for up to 72 hours especially in neonates and infants—watch for respiratory depression. Check cough reflex and ability to swallow. Question any antibiotic orders that prescribe aminoglycosides or tetracycline when neuromuscular blockers have been used.
19. Aminoglycoside antibiotics, beta-adrenergic blocking agents, and diuretics that cause potassium depletion.
20. Anesthesiologist's record

21. See Table 41-2, textbook p. 556.

22. See textbook, p. 555.

23. See textbook, p. 555.

Copyright © 2001 by Mosby, Inc. All rights reserved.

Practice Quiz

Drugs Used to Treat the Muscular System

ESSAY

P.C., age 5 years, is in the postanesthesia recovery area after having abdominal surgery. She received a neuromuscular blocking agent as part of her anesthetic.

1. P.C. is crying with pain, saying, "It hurts!" What additional data should be collected before giving the prescribed analgesic?
2. P.C.'s respirations are 16. What action would you take?
3. Name two muscle relaxants commonly prescribed by physicians in your vicinity and research side effects commonly seen with these agents.
4. What should initial treatment of a musculoskeletal injury include?
5. What is the primary use of centrally acting skeletal muscle relaxants?
6. What premedication assessments are needed for a patient receiving a centrally acting skeletal muscle relaxant?
7. When dantrolene is used to treat neuroleptic malignant syndrome, what baseline assessment is needed?

END-OF-CHAPTER MATH REVIEW

1. Ordered: Methocarbamol (Robaxin) 1.5 g qid
   Convert 1.5 g to _____ mg.

CRITICAL THINKING QUESTIONS

1. D.C. was working in his garden and "pulled a muscle" in his back. The doctor prescribed cyclobenzaprine 10 mg tid for one week. What health teaching should you provide D.C. about the medication and temporary lifestyle changes?
2. Following an extensive major surgical procedure, the patient is transferred to the postanesthesia recovery unit with an endotracheal tube in place. The anesthesia record notes the administration of tubocurarine chloride during the surgical procedure. What criteria should be used to determine when to remove the endotracheal tube? What monitoring of the patient should be done to check for residual effects of the neuromuscular blocking agent?

Copyright © 2001 by Mosby, Inc.   All rights reserved.

CHAPTER CONTENTS

CHAPTER OBJECTIVES

1. Identify significant data in a patient history that could alert the medical team that a patient is more likely to experience an allergic reaction.
2. Identify baseline data the nurse should collect on a continuous basis for comparison and evaluation of antimicrobial drug effectiveness.
3. Describe basic principles of patient care that can be implemented to enhance an individual's therapeutic response during an infection.
4. Identify criteria used to select an effective antimicrobial agent.
5. Differentiate between gram-negative and gram-positive microorganisms and between anaerobic and aerobic properties of microorganisms.
6. Explain the major actions and effects of drugs used to treat infectious diseases.
7. Describe the nursing assessments and interventions for the common side effects associated with antimicrobial agents: allergic reaction; direct tissue damage from nephrotoxicity, ototoxicity, or hepatotoxicity; secondary infection; and other considerations such as photosensitivity, peripheral neuropathy, and neuromuscular blockage.
8. Review techniques and procedures for parenteral administration and vaginal insertion of drugs.
9. Develop an education plan for patients receiving aminoglycosides; cephalosporins; penicillins; quinolones; streptogramins; sulfonamides; tetracyclines; and antitubercular, antifungal, and antiviral agents.

KEY WORDS

pathogenic
antibiotics
nephrotoxicity
ototoxicity
gram-negative
    microorganisms
gram-positive
    microorganisms
hypoprothrombinemia
thrombophlebitis
penicillinase-resistant
    penicillins

ASSIGNMENTS

Read textbook pp. 557-597.
Study Key Words associated with chapter content.
Study Review Sheet for Chapter 43.
Complete End-of-Chapter Math Review and Critical Thinking Questions.
Complete Collaborative Activities as assigned by instructor.
Complete Chapter 43 Practice Quiz.
Complete Chapter 43 Exam.

Copyright © 2001 by Mosby, Inc.   All rights reserved.

COLLABORATIVE ACTIVITIES

Intravenous Antibiotic Therapy

Vancomycin hydrochloride 1 g added to 200 ml 5% D/W to be infused over 60 minutes using an infusion pump calibrated in ml/hr.

1. At what rate should the IV pump be set?
   Run at _____ ml/hr.
2. What premedication assessments should be made prior to the administration of vancomycin hydrochloride?
3. What is "red man syndrome"? What nursing actions should be taken when this occurs?
4. Research the correct procedure for planning or scheduling blood draws for vancomycin serum levels.

Oral Antibiotic Therapy

Zidovudine (AZT) 200 mg po q 4 h is ordered for a patient with acquired immune deficiency syndrome and *Pneumocystis carinii* infection.

1. Explain the desired therapeutic outcome of this drug. Does taking it prevent the transmission of the disease to others?
2. What side effects may occur with the drug's administration and what health teaching should be completed in relation to the administration of this medication?
3. Examine the drug monographs for the antiviral agents used for the treatment of HIV-1.
   a. Do any of the drug monographs state that the use of the drug(s) prevents the spread of HIV through sexual contact or exposure to blood or body secretions?
   b. Which antiviral agents can produce anemia or granulocytopenia?
   c. Which agents can produce confusion?

 Copyright © 2001 by Mosby, Inc.   All rights reserved.

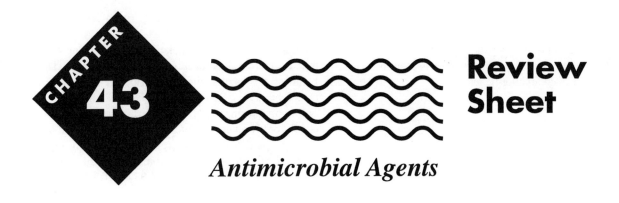

CHAPTER 43

Antimicrobial Agents

Review Sheet

The QUESTION column and the ANSWER column have been offset so that you can cover the answers while reading the questions, allowing you to assess your knowledge.

Question	**Answer**
1. What criteria are used to select an antimicrobial agent?	
2. Describe the signs and symptoms of the common side effects seen with antimicrobial therapy.	1. The physician must choose an antimicrobial agent that will be effective against the type of organism present and one that will not be too toxic to the patient.
	2. Allergy: Rash or skin reaction (e.g., hives with or without dyspnea, laryngeal edema, shock, stridor, and sternal retractions). Direct tissue damage: Hepatotoxicity (liver damage) as noted by an elevation of AST, ALT, GGT, and alkaline phosphatase. Ototoxicity: Dizziness, tinnitus, and progressive hearing loss. Nephrotoxicity (renal damage: as noted by an increase in serum creatinine, BUN, and by alterations in the urine (e.g., decrease in specific gravity, casts, or protein in the urine, and an excess of RBCs over 0 to 3). Secondary infection: Stomatitis, glossitis, itching, vulvovaginitis, cold sores, or canker sores.
3. Differentiate between gram-negative (Gm-) and gram-positive (Gm+) microorganisms, and anaerobic and aerobic properties of microorganisms.	See textbook, p. 559, Blood Dyscrasias, and p. 560, Nausea, Vomiting, and Diarrhea.
4. Describe basic principles of patient care that can be implemented to enhance an individual's therapeutic response during an infection.	3. Classification of microorganisms as gram-positive or gram-negative refers to the type of staining properties of a bacterium. Cells with a cell wall retain stain and are referred to as gram+ cells. Cells without a cell wall do not retain the gram stain, and are referred to as gram- cells. Broad spectrum antibiotics are effective against many gram-positive and gram-negative organisms. Anaerobic bacteria grow in the absence of oxygen; aerobic bacteria require oxygen to reproduce.
5. Review components of a baseline assessment to evaluate a patient's hydration status and assessments needed to detect renal or hepatic toxicity.	4. Adequate rest, hydration, and nutrients. Teach personal hygiene measures, (e.g., hand washing, proper techniques for changing dressings).

Copyright © 2001 by Mosby, Inc. All rights reserved.

6. Identify significant data in a patient's history that could alert the medical team that the patient is more likely to experience an allergic reaction.

7. Describe the usual management of nausea, vomiting, and diarrhea when they occur in conjunction with antimicrobial therapy.

8. State the signs and symptoms of a secondary infection and actions that can be taken to minimize these effects.

9. Review techniques and procedures for parenteral administration and vaginal insertion of drugs.

10. Identify significant information relating to patient education when caring for a person receiving an antibiotic.

11. Cite the primary uses of aminoglycosides and the serious side effects that require close monitoring of the patient.

12. Identify precautions needed to prevent incompatibilities between aminoglycosides and other medications.

13. State the mechanism of action of aminoglycosides on the bacterial cell.

14. What premedication assessments should be made before aminoglycoside therapy?

15. Cite the effectiveness of cephalosporins, according to generation, against gram-positive and gram-negative microorganisms.

5. Hydration: Skin turgor, intake and output, inspect mucous membranes for moisture or dryness, check firmness of eyeballs, check specific gravity of urine (see Table 39-1). Renal toxicity: Decreasing urine output, increasing BUN and/or serum creatinine; check for presence of protein, blood, or casts in the urine. Hepatic toxicity: Anorexia, nausea, vomiting, jaundice, hepatomegaly, splenomegaly, and abnormal (elevated) liver function tests (AST, ALT, LDH, GGT alkaline phosphatase).

6. Before administering any antibiotic, check for any prior allergies to medications or foods or the presence of asthma. If the patient is allergic to anything, get details regarding the symptoms and previous treatment of the allergy.

7. Gather data relative to the patient's usual pattern of elimination (e.g., number of stools per day, consistency) and compare this information with the current data. Read individual drug monographs to identify antimicrobials that may cause diarrhea, nausea, or vomiting. Report these to the physician.

8. Be particularly alert for secondary infection in patients receiving broad spectrum antibiotics and those patients who are immunosuppressed. Assess for white patches in the mouth, cold sores, canker sores, vaginal itching, diarrhea, and recurrent fever.

9. See Chapter 9, Parenteral Administration and Chapter 10, Percutaneous Administration.

10. With the instructor's assistance, identify significant points relating to the prescribed drug therapy that should be taught to the patient for each class of antimicrobials ordered.

11. Aminoglycosides are used to treat gram-negative bacteria causing meningitis, wound infections, chronic urinary tract infections, and life-threatening septicemia. Monitor the patient closely for ototoxicity and nephrotoxicity.

12. Do not mix aminoglycosides in the same syringe or infuse these drugs simultaneously with other medications. Tag the chart of any patient going to surgery who is receiving an aminoglycoside. Respiratory depression may occur when these agents are combined with skeletal muscle relaxants.

13. Aminoglycosides inhibit protein synthesis of bacteria.

14. Baseline assessment of allergies, presenting symptoms, T, P, R, BP, and hydration status. Check for any hearing disorders or deficits or renal disease. If present, hold drug and notify physician. Check for patient having received any skeletal muscle relaxants within the past 72 hours. If taking aminoglycosides, check serum level. Check for laboratory results ordered by the physician (e.g., CBC with differential).

Copyright © 2001 by Mosby, Inc. All rights reserved.

16. What premedication assessments should be performed before therapy with cephalosporins?

15. The first generation cephalosporins have good activity against gram-positive bacteria and mild activity against gram-negative bacteria. The second generation cephalosporins have somewhat increased activity against gram-negative bacteria but are much less active than the third generation agents. The third generation agents are less active than first generation agents against gram-positive cocci. Some of the third generation agents are also active against *Pseudomonas aeruginosa*, a very potent gram-negative microorganism. The third generation cephalosporins have greater activity against gram-positive penicillinase-producing bacteria than first generation cephalosporins. Fourth generation cephalosporins are considered broad spectrum, with both gram-negative and gram-positive coverage.

17. State the mechanism of action of cephalosporins on the cell wall.

16. Baseline assessment of allergies, presenting symptoms, T, P, R, BP, and hydration status, symptoms of renal disease or bleeding disorder (hold drug and notify physician if present), and laboratory studies as ordered by physician (e.g., CBC with differential).

18. What types of infections can be treated effectively using cephalosporins?

17. Interferes with synthesis of bacterial cell wall.

19. What side effects from cephalosporins should be reported?

18. Respiratory, urinary, gastrointestinal, skin, and soft tissue infections, septicemia, meningitis, osteomyelitis, and certain sexually transmitted diseases

20. Why may hypoprothrombinemia occur with cephalosporin therapy?

19. Diarrhea, secondary infections, abnormal liver and renal function tests

21. What are the signs and symptoms of thrombophlebitis, which may occur with cephalosporin therapy?

20. Although rare, hypoprothrombinemia may develop in the elderly, debilitated, or otherwise compromised patient with borderline vitamin K deficiency. Treatment with broad spectrum antibiotics eliminates enough gastrointestinal flora to cause a further reduction in vitamin K synthesis.

22. What precautions should be instituted when cephalosporins are combined with probenecid or alcohol?

21. Report redness, warmth, tenderness to touch, or edema in the affected part. Homan's sign in lower extremities.

23. What is the difference between bacteriostatic and bacteriocidal?

22. Probenecid with cephalosporins may increase likelihood of toxicity. When combined with alcohol, cephalosporins may produce flushing, dyspnea, tachycardia, and hypotension. Do not ingest alcohol within 72 hours of taking cephalosporins.

24. Identify the uses of macrolides.

23. Bacteriocidal agents kill the microorganism; bacteriostatic agents weaken the microorganism. Whether an agent is bacteriostatic or bacteriocidal depends on the organism and concentration of medication present.

24. Macrolides are used for respiratory, gastrointestinal tract, skin, and soft tissue infections and STDs, especially when penicillins, cephalosporins, and tetracyclines cannot be used.

25. State the actions of penicillins on the bacterial cell.

25. Penicillins act by interfering with the synthesis of the bacterial cell wall. They are most effective against bacteria that are multiplying.

26. Identify the clinical uses of penicillins.

Copyright © 2001 by Mosby, Inc. All rights reserved.

27. For what types of adverse effects should a patient taking penicillin be monitored?

28. Cite questions that should be asked to screen a patient for a penicillin allergy before administration of the agent.

29. Identify precautions necessary to prevent an incompatibility between penicillin and other medications given intramuscularly or intravenously.

30. Briefly describe the mechanisms of action of the quinolones and fluroquinolones and list the uses of these agents.

31. Review the multiple uses of quinolones and fluroquinolones.

32. Why are the quinolones are not used in children under the age of 12 years?

33. What premedication assessments should be made prior to beginning quinolone therapy?

34. Describe the effects of antacids, iron, and sucralfate on quinolones and the adaptations in scheduling required if both agents are prescribed concurrently.

35. What is the mechanism of action of the new class of antibiotics known as streptogramins?

36. What are the uses of streptogramins?

37. What precautions need to be used when reconstituting streptogramins or administering them IV?

38. Cite the mechanism of action of sulfonamides and the importance of monitoring following administration.

39. State the effect of sulfonamides on persons taking sulfonylurea oral hypoglycemic agents.

26. Treatment of middle ear infection, pneumonia, meningitis, urinary tract infections, syphilis, and gonorrhea; and as a prophylactic antibiotic before surgery or dental procedures for patients with a history of rheumatic fever.

27. Watch for diarrhea, abnormal liver and renal function tests, thrombophlebitis, and electrolyte imbalances from sodium or potassium types of penicillin. Elderly or debilitated patients with impaired renal function are more likely to develop adverse effects.

28. "Have you ever taken an antibiotic before? Do you have any known allergies to foods or medications?" If so, obtain further details, such as: "When you got sick while taking the medication, what symptoms did you have? What did the doctor tell you to do when this occurred? Do you have hay fever or asthma?"

29. Do not mix penicillin with other drugs in the same syringe or infuse together with other drugs.

30. Quinolones act by interfering with replication of bacterial DNA. Quinolones are effective against gram-negative and gram-positive bacteria, including anaerobes. Fluroquinolones act by inhibiting activity of DNA gyrase, an enzyme essential for the replication of bacterial DNA.

31. See textbook p. 568.

32. Quinolones may cause permanent damage to cartilage in a pediatric patient.

33. Baseline assessment of allergies, presenting symptoms, T, P, R, BP, and hydration status, gastric symptoms present, baseline laboratory studies as ordered, check for pregnancy. Warn about possible photosensitivity with lomefloxacin.

34. Antacids, iron-containing products, and sucralfate may decrease the absorption of quinolones. The antibiotic should be scheduled 4 hours before or 4 hours after taking any of these medications.

35. Streptogramins (quinupristin, dalfopristin) act by inhibiting protein synthesis in bacterial cell wall.

36. These agents should be reserved for treatment of serious or life-threatening infections associated with vancomycin resistance.

37. See textbook p. 571.

38. Sulfonamides inhibit bacterial biosynthesis of folic acid, leading to inadequate metabolism and cell death. Persons taking sulfonamides for 14 days or more need periodic monitoring of RBC and WBC (with differential) counts. All patients receiving sulfonamides need adequate hydration and should be encouraged to drink eight 12 oz glasses of water daily.

Copyright © 2001 by Mosby, Inc.   All rights reserved.

40. State the mechanism of action of tetracyclines.

41. List a minimum of two types of antibiotics that may cause photosensitivity.
42. Identify the effects of administering tetracyclines during pregnancy and at the age of tooth development.

43. Describe the dosage and administration considerations when tetracycline is prescribed.

44. Identify the causative organism and mode of transfer of tuberculosis.

45. Describe factors that need consideration to enhance a patient's response to antitubercular therapy.

46. Develop a teaching plan for persons receiving antitubercular agents.

47. Compare the mechanisms of action of ethambutol, isoniazid, and rifampin.
48. Identify the effects of rifampin on body secretions (e.g., urine, feces, saliva, and sputum).

49. What is the mechanism of action of monobactams?

50. What is the mechanism of action of chloramphenicol?

51. State specific limitations for the use of chloramphenicol.
52. Identify specific nursing assessments needed to detect possible serious hematologic effects from chloramphenicol.

39. Sulfonamides may displace sulfonylurea oral hypoglycemic agents from their protein binding sites, potentially resulting in hypoglycemia. Have patients taking these two agents concurrently test their blood glucose or urine 1/2 hour ac and hs to detect the development of a problem.
40. Tetracyclines inhibit protein synthesis by bacterial cells.
41. Quinolones, tetracyclines, sulfonamides, and griseofulvin may cause photosensitivity. Patients taking these antibiotics should be cautioned to avoid exposure to sunlight and ultraviolet lights. Discourage the use of artificial tanning lights and instruct patients to wear clothing that provides adequate coverage of the body when in the sunlight.
42. Do not administer tetracycline during the last half of pregnancy or to children through 8 years of age because it may cause enamel hypoplasia and permanent staining of the teeth. Do not administer to nursing mothers because it is secreted in breast milk.
43. Take medication 1 hour before or 2 hours after ingesting antacids; milk; dairy products; or products containing calcium, aluminum, magnesium (antacids), or iron (vitamins).
Exception: Doxycycline is not affected by food or milk.
44. *Mycobacterium tuberculosis* is spread by airborne droplets from the cough or sneeze of a person infected with the organism.
45. Personal hygiene, nutritional status, and stress reduction are factors that must be considered during the treatment of tuberculosis.
46. Review your teaching plan with the course instructor.
47. Ethambutol inhibits TB bacterial growth by altering cellular RNA synthesis and phosphate metabolism. The mechanism of action of isoniazid is unknown. It appears to disrupt the *M. tuberculosis* cell wall and inhibit replication. Rifampin acts against enzymes in the bacterial cell required to produce DNA.
48. Rifampin may tinge urine, feces, saliva, sweat, and tears a reddish-orange color.
49. Monobactams are a new class of synthetic, bacteriocidal antibiotics that act by inhibiting cell wall synthesis.
50. Chloramphenicol acts by inhibiting bacterial protein synthesis.
51. Use only for serious infections; it is particularly effective in treating rickettsial infections, meningitis, and typhoid fever.

Copyright © 2001 by Mosby, Inc.   All rights reserved.

53. What is the mechanism of action of clindamycin?

54. Describe effective treatment for diarrhea associated with clindamycin therapy.
55. Identify the mechanism of action and the primary therapeutic use of imipenem/cilastatin.

56. State precautions and specific data that should be sought from the patient before initiating the administration of imipenem/cilastatin.

57. Summarize baseline assessments needed to evaluate a patient's mental status and specific seizure precautions that should be implemented when imipenem/cilastatin therapy is initiated.
58. Identify the specific intravenous recommendations associated with intravenous infusion of imipenem/cilastatin.

59. State the primary clinical uses for metronidazole.

60. What is the mechanism of action of spectinomycin?

61. Identify the effectiveness of spectinomycin against gonorrhea and syphilis.
62. Cite specific recommendations for intramuscular administration of spectinomycin.

63. Why should serology testing for syphilis be done prior to initiating therapy using spectinomycin?

64. What is the mechanism of action of vancomycin?
65. Describe nursing assessments that may be used to detect ototoxicity.
66. Describe "red man syndrome" and identify the drug is associated with its occurrence.

67. What type of dressings should be avoided with topical antifungal medications and what type of precautions should be taken to prevent accidental pregnancy when these drugs are administered intravaginally?

52. Check for sore throat, feelings of fatigue, elevated temperature, small petechial hemorrhages, and bruises of the skin. Report any of these symptoms immediately to the physician. Routine laboratory studies including RBC, WBC, and differential counts are scheduled for patients taking chloramphenicol 14 days or longer.
53. Clindamycin acts by inhibiting protein synthesis.

54. Do not self-treat diarrhea. (Kaopectate for persistent diarrhea from clindamycin therapy is used since it absorbs clindamycin. Do not use diphenoxylate, loperamide, or paregoric.)
Patients should be instructed to contact the physician for specific directions and not to self-treat the diarrhea.
55. Imipenem/cilastatin is used to treat severe infections caused by multiresistant organisms and mixed anaerobic/aerobic infections, primarily those involving intra-abdominal and pelvic sepsis. It acts by inhibiting bacterial cell wall synthesis.
56. Screen for allergies to penicillin or cephalosporins.

57. Check for a history of seizures before initiating imipenem/cilastatin. Check patient's orientation to date, time, place, and appropriateness of responses to situations or questions asked before initiation of therapy and at regular intervals thereafter.
58. Check for signs and symptoms of phlebitis during IV administration of imipenem/cilastatin. See specific directions for reconstitution and IV administration, p. 579.
59. Metronidazole is used to treat trichomoniasis, giardiasis, amebic dysentery, amebic liver abscess, and anaerobic bacterial infections.
60. Spectinomycin acts by inhibiting protein synthesis.

61. Spectinomycin is used to treat gonorrhea in both males and females. It is not effective in treatment of syphilis.
62. Use a 20 gauge needle, and inject into upper outer quadrant of gluteal muscle. Causes pain at injection site.
63. This drug masks symptoms of syphilis.
64. Vancomycin acts by preventing synthesis of bacterial cell wall.
65. Dizziness, tinnitus, and progressive hearing loss (e.g., turns the TV on louder, has to have conversation repeated).
66. Red man syndrome or redneck syndrome is caused by rapid IV infusion of vancomycin; symptoms include sudden hypotension with or without maculopapular rash over face, neck, upper chest, and extremities.

Copyright © 2001 by Mosby, Inc.   All rights reserved.

68. What is the mechanism of action of amphotericin B?

69. Cite the primary uses of amphotericin B.

70. Describe the systemic side effects seen with intravenous administration of amphotericin B.

71. Identify the monitoring parameters used to detect nephrotoxicity.

72. Cite specific dosage and administration characteristics associated with the use of amphotericin B.

73. Describe the effects of light on amphotericin B.
74. List medications that may occasionally be added to amphotericin B suspensions to minimize venous irritation.
75. Review procedures used to administer topical medications to the skin.

76. Describe the uses of fluconazole (Diflucan) and flucytosine (Ancobon, Ancotil).
77. Describe the mechanisms of action and uses of griseofulvin (Fulvicin, Grifulvin).

78. State laboratory tests needed periodically to monitor renal, hepatic, and hematopoietic function when griseofulvin is administered.
79. State the mechanisms of action and types of fungal infections for which itraconazole, ketoconazole, miconazole, and terbinafine are used.

67. Avoid occlusive dressings. Alternative forms of birth control should also be used when antifungal ointments are instilled intravaginally. Diaphragms and condoms may deteriorate with prolonged contact with petroleum-based ointment.
68. Amphotericin B disrupts the cell membrane of fungal cells resulting in loss of cellular content and death of the cell.
69. Amphotericin B is used to treat systemic fungal infections and meningitis. Topically, it can be used for candidal infections.
70. Nephrotoxicity, electrolyte imbalances, chills, fever, malaise, headache, nausea and vomiting, and thrombophlebitis.
71. Nephrotoxicity is indicated by increased excretion of uric acid, magnesium, oliguria, granular casts in urine, proteinuria, increased BUN, and serum creatinine. Report decrease in daily urine volume or changes in visual appearance of the urine.
72. See textbook, pp. 584-585.
73. Amphotericin B deteriorates in the presence of light. Cover the solution to protect it from light during administration.
74. Heparin, hydrocortisone, or methylprednisolone may be added to infusion solution to diminish venous irritation.
75. See chapter 10, Percutaneous Medications.

76. Fluconazole is used for cryptococcal meningitis and oropharyngeal, esophageal, vulvovaginal or systemic candidiasis. Flucytosine is effective against susceptible candidal septicemia, endocarditis, urinary tract infections, cryptococcal meningitis, and pulmonary infections.
77. Griseofulvin acts by stopping cell division and new cell growth and is used to treat ringworm of scalp, body, nails, and feet.
78. Hepatotoxicity (liver damage) is noted by an elevation in AST, ALT, GGT, and alkaline phosphatase. Nephrotoxicity (renal damage) is indicated by an increase in serum creatinine, BUN, and by alterations in the urine (e.g., decrease in specific gravity, casts or protein in the urine, and an excess of RBCs over 0 to 3). Hematologic: Monitor for the development of sore throat, fever, purpura, jaundice, or excessive progressive weakness.

Copyright © 2001 by Mosby, Inc. All rights reserved.

80. Identify the mechanism of action of acyclovir, didanosine, famiciclovir, and valacyclovir.

81. Cite the potential effects of acyclovir on renal function.
82. Identify the first antiviral agent that is effective against respiratory viruses.

83. Cite the clinical limitations of zidovudine in the treatment of HIV (human immunodeficiency virus).
84. Identify the hematologic tests that should be completed periodically during the use of zidovudine.

85. Describe the effect of zidovudine on transmission of HIV to others through sexual contact or blood contamination.
86. Describe the proper schedule for administering zidovudine and essential health teaching needed.

87. Review current Centers for Disease Control recommendations for handling body secretions and blood for all patients.
88. Which of the antiviral agents may reduce pulmonary function?

89. Which antiviral agent may reduce the effectiveness of oral contraceptives?
90. Which antiviral agents may produce peripheral neuropathy?
91. Study the antibiotic tables throughout the chapter and identify common endings in the generic names of the antimicrobial agents.

79. Ketoconazole, itraconazole, and miconazole act by interfering with cell wall synthesis, causing leakage of cellular contents. (Terbinafine, see textbook pp. 588-589.) Ketoconazole is used orally to treat candidiasis, chronic mucocutaneous candidiasis, oral thrush, coccidioidomycosis, histoplasmosis, chromomycosis, and paracoccidioidomycosis. Miconazole is used parenterally to treat similar fungal infections. Terbinafine is used to treat onychomycosis of the toenail or fingernail due to dermatophytes. (Itraconazole, see textbook pp. 587-588.)

80. These antiviral agents act by inhibiting the viral cell wall replication.
81. Transient elevation of serum creatinine. Patients who are poorly hydrated, have low renal function, or who receive acyclovir by a bolus are susceptible to renal tubular damage.
82. Ribavirin (Virazole)

83. It prolongs the lives of AIDS and ARC patients, reduces the risk and severity of opportunistic infections, and improves immune status. Zidovudine does not cure acquired immunodeficiency.
84. Monitor CBC with differential, platelets, hemoglobin, hematocrit, amylase, and liver function tests.

85. This drug does not reduce the risk of transmitting HIV to others through sexual contact or blood contamination.
86. Oral medication is taken every 4 hours around the clock even though it interrupts normal sleep. Do not share with other persons.
87. Check with your instructor to obtain the latest recommendations or research the information on the CDC website.
88. Both ribavirin and zanamivir may affect pulmonary function.
89. Amprenavir

90. Didanosine, lamivudine, zidovudine

91. See textbook Tables 43-1 through 43-8.

Copyright © 2001 by Mosby, Inc.   All rights reserved.

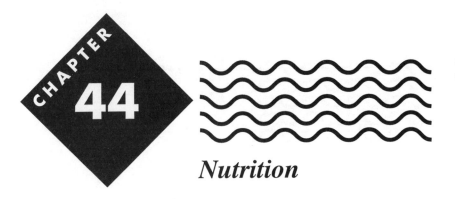

CHAPTER 44

Nutrition

Syllabus

CHAPTER CONTENTS

Principles of Nutrition (p. 599)
Malnutrition (p. 604)
Therapy for Malnutrition (p. 605)

CHAPTER OBJECTIVES

1. Differentiate between information found in the dietary reference intake tables and the recommended dietary allowance tables.
2. Identify the function of macronutrients in the body.
3. State the formula used to estimate basal energy expenditures for males and females.
4. Differentiate between fat-soluble and water-soluble vitamins.
5. List five functions of minerals in the body.
6. Describe nutritional assessments essential prior to administration of tube feedings and parenteral nutrition.
7. Describe physical changes associated with a malnourished state.
8. Cite common laboratory and diagnostic tests used to monitor a patient's nutritional status.
9. Discuss nursing assessments and interventions required during the administration of enteral nutrition.
10. Discuss home care needs of a patient being discharged on any form of enteral or parenteral nutrition.

KEY WORDS

dietary reference intakes
    (DRI)
recommended dietary
    allowances (RDA)
adequate intake (AI)
estimated average
    requirement (EAR)
tolerable upper intake
    level (UL)
kilocalories

carbohydrate
monosaccharides
disaccharides
fats
lipids
proteins
glucogenesis
vitamins
minerals
water

marasmus
kwashiorkor
mixed kwashiorkor-
    marasmus
enteral nutrition

tube feedings
hyperalimentation
total parenteral nutrition
    (TPN)

ASSIGNMENTS

Read textbook pages 599-612.
Study Key Words associated with the chapter content.
Study Review Sheet for Chapter 44.
Complete End-of-Chapter Math Review and Critical Thinking Questions.
Complete Collaborative Activities as assigned by instructor.
Complete Chapter 44 Practice Quiz.
Complete Chapter 44 Exam.

COLLABORATIVE ACTIVITIES

Answer the following questions. Be prepared to share your answers during in-class discussion and group work that may be assigned by the instructor.

1. Use a laboratory reference book to research the normal findings for the following lab tests used to assess lean body mass: albumin, prealbumin, retinol-binding protein, and transferrin.
2. Research the policy used at the clinical site where you are assigned for checking feeding tube placement and residual volumes.
3. Review the procedure manual at your clinical site to determine the procedure for monitoring total parenteral nutrition (TPN) (hyperalimentation).
4. Review the drug interactions listed for enteral and parenteral nutrition products.

Copyright © 2001 by Mosby, Inc.   All rights reserved.

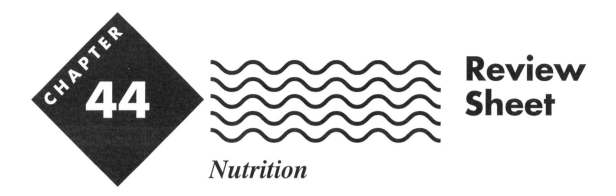

The QUESTION column and the ANSWER column have been offset so that you can cover the answers while reading the questions, allowing you to assess your knowledge.

Question	**Answer**
1. What factors affect one's nutritional requirements?	
2. What information can be found in the Dietary Reference Intake (DRI) table and Recommended Dietary Allowance (RDA) table?	1. See textbook, p. 599.
3. What is the unit of measurement of energy requirements?	2. See Table 44-1 and textbook p. 600.
4. What does the Harris-Benedict equation calculate?	3. Kilocalories (kcal)
5. What are other names for simple carbohydrates?	4. The Harris-Benedict equation is one approach to calculating the total calories needed.
6. State the daily caloric needs from carbohydrates required.	5. Simple carbohydrates are known as monosaccharides and disaccharides.
7. Carbohydrates supply _____ kilocalories of energy per gram, fats supply _____ kilocalories of energy per gram, and proteins supply _____ kilocalories of energy per gram.	6. Range is from 3 to 5.5 grams/kg/day, depending on energy requirements for daily living, stress, and wound healing.
8. What are the end products of protein metabolism?	7. Carbohydrates supply 4 kilocalories, fats supply 9 kilocalories, and proteins supply 4 kilocalories.
9. How many water-soluble and fat-soluble vitamins are there to date?	8. Nitrogenous products such as urea, uric acid, ammonium, carbon dioxide, and water.
10. Name the three types of malnutrition.	9. Thirteen total vitamins; 9 water-soluble; 4 fat-soluble.
11. What laboratory studies can be used to assess lean body mass?	10. Marasmus, kwashiorkor, and mixed kwashiorkor-marasmus
12. Differentiate between enteral and parenteral nutrition.	11. Albumin, prealbumin, retinol-binding protein, transferrin
13. Explain components of a nutritional assessment.	12. Enteral nutrition is administered orally; parenteral nutrition is given via venous access and implantable vascular access devices.
14. What physical changes are related to a malnourished state?	13. See textbook, pp. 605-606.
15. What are the general routines used for checking tube placement and residuals?	14. Height, weight, muscle circumference, skin fold thickness, skin integrity, cardiovascular, respiratory, neurological alteration, thyroid function, gastrointestinal symptoms.
16. When is the use of enteral nutrition contraindicated?	15. See textbook, p. 606.

Copyright © 2001 by Mosby, Inc.   All rights reserved.

17. What premedication assessments should be performed prior to administering enteral nutrition?

18. Differentiate between bolus, intermittent, and continuous feedings.
19. How should prescribed medications be administered via a feeding tube?
20. List side effects of enteral feedings that should be reported to the physician.
21. Review the drug monograph for enteral nutrition and note drugs that interact with grapefruit juice.

22. What is the difference between total parenteral nutrition, peripheral parenteral nutrition solutions (PPN), and total parenteral nutrition (TPN) solutions?
23. List premedication assessments that should be performed before administering TPN or PPN.

24. List side effects of parenteral feedings that should be reported to the physician.
25. List key signs and symptoms of fat-soluble and water-soluble vitamin deficiencies.

16. Enteral nutrition is contraindicated when the individual has intractable vomiting, a paralyzed ileum, or certain types of fistulas.
17. See textbook, p. 608.

18. See textbook, p. 609.

19. See textbook, pp. 609-610.

20. Pulmonary complications (aspiration), diarrhea, constipation, nausea, vomiting, increased residual volume, rash, chills, fever, and respiratory difficulty.
21. See textbook, p. 610.

22. PPN solutions consist of 2% to 5% crystalline amino acid preparations and 5% to 10% dextrose with electrolytes and vitamins. TPN consists of 15% to 25% glucose, amino acids (3.5 to 15%), fat emulsion (10% to 20%), electrolytes, vitamins and minerals.
23. See textbook, p. 611.

24. Hypoglycemia, hyperglycemia , fluid imbalance, rash, chills, fever, respiratory difficulty, electrolyte imbalances, and hepatotoxicity
25. See textbook, p. 603.

Copyright © 2001 by Mosby, Inc. All rights reserved.

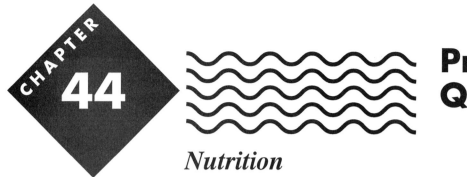

CHAPTER 44

Nutrition

Practice Quiz

TRUE OR FALSE

Mark each statement "T" for true and "F" for false.
<u>*Correct all false statements.*</u>

_____ 1. The recommended dietary allowance (RDA) table contains a listing of the average dietary intake sufficient for the nutritional requirements of an adult with active disease process present.

_____ 2. The Harris-Benedict equation is used to calculate the amount of carbohydrates needed daily in the diet.

_____ 3. The daily carbohydrate needs are 1 to 1.5 grams/kg/day.

_____ 4. Carbohydrates and proteins supply approximately 4 kilocalories of energy per gram.

_____ 5. The fat-soluble vitamins are D, E, A, and K.

_____ 6. Kwashiorkor is a protein deficiency resulting from a diet that provides adequate carbohydrate and fats, but insufficient protein.

_____ 7. From research on assigned laboratory studies it is apparent that a decreased albumin level is related to the maintenance of oncotic pressure in the vascular system.

_____ 8. Prealbumin is an indicator of recent catabolism in the body.

_____ 9. Osmolyte is an example of a total parenteral nutrition (TPN) formula.

_____ 10. Edema of the abdomen and subcutaneous tissue is a possible sign of protein deficiency.

_____ 11. A thiamine deficiency can increase the heart rate and heart size.

_____ 12. Stomach content residuals from tube feedings are generally checked prior to each bolus feeding and once every 24 hours for continuous enteral feedings.

_____ 13. During hyperalimentation, the client is generally placed on insulin by sliding scale.

_____ 14. Prior to hanging a TPN solution, two qualified nurses should check the contents of the container against the specific doctor's order.

_____ 15. Special enteral feeding formulas are available for persons with hepatic, renal, pulmonary, or malabsorption syndromes.

_____ 16. The enteral feeding tube should be clamped 30 to 60 minutes before administering a prescribed medication that should be taken on an empty stomach.

_____ 17. Persons receiving tube feedings should have the head of the bed (HOB) elevated 45 degrees on a continuous basis.

_____ 18. TPN consists of a parenteral nutrition solution that is 2% to 5% crystalline amino acids, and 5% to 10% dextrose with added electrolytes and vitamins.

_____ 19. TPN solutions can be given directly via an IV administration set.

_____ 20. A pyridoxine deficiency can result in anemia, dyspnea, cardiomegaly, and heart failure.

_____ 21. Vitamin C deficiency can result in anemia, depression, and delayed wound healing.

_____ 22. Intravenous lines used to administer TPN may be used for the administration of multiple medications simultaneously with the parenteral feeding.

_____ 23. Signs and symptoms of dehydration or overhydration should be monitored on a continuum during enteral and parenteral nutritional therapy.

Copyright © 2001 by Mosby, Inc.   All rights reserved.

END-OF-CHAPTER MATH REVIEW

1. M.B. has an order to receive Osmolyte, full strength, at 80 ml per hour around the clock. The feeding is shut off for an hour 3 times per day when medications are administered that interact with the nutritional product. What adjustments in the rate of administration should be made to administer the full amount of prescribed formula during the hours it is running?
2. A client is receiving intermittent bolus feedings of Ensure 250 cc every 4 hours, followed by a water bolus of 150 ml per feeding. What is the individual's total fluid intake over a 24-hour period?

CRITICAL THINKING QUESTIONS

1. A client's TPN solution has gotten behind in the rate of administration. As the nurse, you realize the client needs the nutrients. What interventions could be initiated and what actions would be contraindicated? Give your rationale.

2. In a nursing home the client on a continuous tube feeding could have the tube feeding scheduled to run at night, allowing greater mobility during the daytime. If the client needs an intake of 80 ml per hour over a 24-hour time span, how would the hourly intake be adjusted to administer the enteral product between 8 PM and 8 AM?
3. Explain teaching you would institute for an adult being discharged on bolus enteral feedings. How would you teach the person to administer the enteral product and what monitoring for complications should be done prior to discharge?
4. It is time to hang the next bag of TPN and it has not arrived from the pharmacy. What would be appropriate actions for the nurse to take?
5. While caring for an elderly client receiving continuous tube feedings using a kangaroo feeding pump, you suspect the patient has aspirated some of the formula. What symptoms would you assess for and what immediate nursing actions should you take?

Copyright © 2001 by Mosby, Inc. All rights reserved.

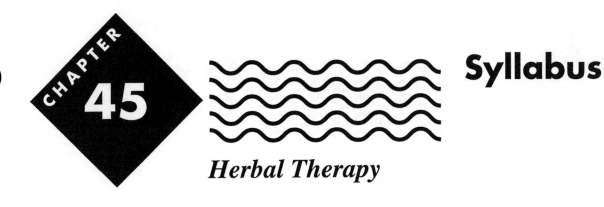

CHAPTER 45

Herbal Therapy

Syllabus

CHAPTER CONTENTS

Herbal Medicines (p. 613)
Drug Therapy (p. 615)
    Black Cohosh (p. 615)
    Chamomile (p. 615)
    Echinacea (p. 615)
    Ephedra (p. 616)
    Feverfew (p. 616)
    Garlic (p. 617)
    Ginkgo (p. 617)
    Ginseng (p. 617)
    Goldenseal (p. 618)
    Saw Palmetto (p. 618)
    St. John's Wort (p. 619)
    Valerian (p. 619)

CHAPTER OBJECTIVES

1. Summarize the primary actions, uses, and interactions of the herbal products listed.
2. Describe the possible impact of the use of herbal products on cultural or ethnic beliefs.

KEY WORDS

herbal medicines
botanicals
phytomedicine
phytotherapy

ASSIGNMENTS

Read textbook pp. 613-620.
Study Key Words associated with chapter content.
Study Review Sheet for Chapter 45.
Complete End-of-Chapter Math Review and Critical Thinking Questions.
Complete Collaborative Activities as assigned by instructor.
Complete Chapter 45 Practice Quiz.
Complete Chapter 45 Exam.

COLLABORATIVE ACTIVITIES

Complete the following as preparation for in-class discussion and group work that may be assigned by the instructor.

1. Go to a health food store that sells herbal products and have the salesperson recommend some products for the treatment of depression, lack of energy, and general malaise. Ask the salesperson about his or her background or qualifications to make these recommendations.
2. Research the herbal products available at a drug store and their cost (e.g., St. John's Wort).
3. Research cultural beliefs regarding herbal products.
4. Check for the resources available on herbal products at the clinical unit where you are assigned.

Copyright © 2001 by Mosby, Inc.   All rights reserved.

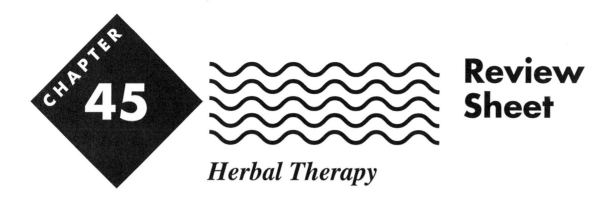

Herbal Therapy

The QUESTION column and the ANSWER column have been offset so that you can cover the answers while reading the questions, allowing you to assess your knowledge.

Question	Answer
1. Define the key words associated with this chapter.	1. See textbook, pp. 613.
2. Describe the role of the Food and Drug Administration (FDA) in the regulation of herbal products.	2. The FDA has no direct role in regulation of herbal products. The Dietary Supplement Health and Education Act (DSHEA) of 1994 governs the use of herbal medicines, vitamins, minerals, and amino acids.
3. Study Box 45-1 for factors to be considered when recommending herbal products.	3. See Box 45-1, p. 614.
4. Develop questions for use as part of a medication history that would elicit information regarding the use of herbal products and other alternative medicines.	4. See your instructor for assistance.
5. Develop a list of the actions and potential drug interactions for each herbal product discussed.	5. See individual herbal monographs throughout chapter.

    Copyright © 2001 by Mosby, Inc.   All rights reserved.

Practice Quiz

Herbal Therapy

ESSAY

1. Define *herbal medicine, botanicals, phytomedicine,* and *phytotherapy.*
2. Describe legal and ethical dilemmas associated with herbal products for nurses, doctors, and other health care workers.
3. Discuss the following statement made by a patient: "The only thing I've been using for medications are harmless herbal products I purchase at my pharmacy."
4. Use the textbook to prepare a list of the herbal products and the associated actions of each, emphasizing drug interactions that may occur with herbal products.

COMPLETION

Complete the following statements.

5. Black cohosh interacts with _____ medications.
6. Echinacea is an _____ system stimulator.
7. Garlic is primarily used for _____.
8. The herbal product used for symptoms of benign prostatic hyperplasia is _____.

CRITICAL THINKING QUESTIONS

1. Discuss the pros and cons of allowing a patient to use herbal products for self-treatment of such things as premenstrual syndrome (black cohash), especially if the woman is using an estrogen/progestin replacement therapy hormone as well. What if the individual also has hypertension?
2. What recommendations should a nurse make to an immunocompromised patient who asks about taking echinacea as an anti-inflammatory agent for "arthritis"?
3. Research the law in the state where you reside with regard to the use of ephedrine.
4. What health teaching should be done for a patient taking nonsteroidal anti-inflammatory agents and feverfew concurrently?
5. What herbal products listed in this chapter interact with anticoagulants?

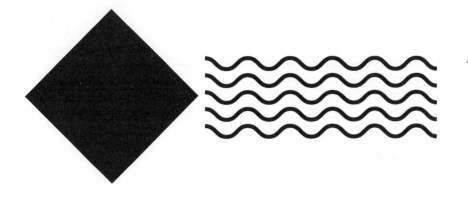

Answers

CHAPTER 1

1. pharmacology
2. drug
3. The chemical name describes the exact placement of atoms and molecular groupings of a chemical compound; it is of most value to the chemist. The brand name, also known as the trade name, is used by a particular manufacturer to market a drug. The brand name is capitalized and is followed by an ®, which is the symbol of a registered trademark. The generic name is given to a drug and is used as the official name for reference to the drug by any and all manufacturers and in all countries. It is not capitalized.
4. Brand names: Bayer®, Ecotrin®, Empirin®
   Generic name: aspirin
5. Brand names: Anacin-3®, Datril®, Tempra®, Tylenol®
   Generic name: acetaminophen
6. Brand name: Pepto-Bismol®
   Generic names: bismuth subsalicylate
7. Brand names: Maalox®, Gelusil II®, Aludrox®
   Generic name ingredients: magnesium hydroxide and aluminum hydroxide
8. Brand names: Motrin IB®, Advil®, Nuprin®
   Generic name: ibuprofen
9. Brand names: Tums®, Bio-Cal®, Cal-Sup®
   Generic name: calcium carbonate

10. *American Drug Index*: Index for all drugs available in U.S.
11. *American Hospital Formulary Service, Drug Information*: Contains drug monographs on every single-drug entity available in U.S.
12. *Facts and Comparisons*: Book is arranged by body systems. Each chapter is subdivided by therapeutic classes. The data in each monograph is the most current FDA-approved package insert information and includes publication from official groups; e.g., CDC and National Academy of Science.
13. *Martindale—The Complete Drug Reference*: Comprehensive text of drugs used throughout the world.
14. *Handbook of Nonprescription Drugs*: Most comprehensive book on medicines sold over-the-counter in the United States.
15. *Medical Letter*: A biweekly newsletter with comments on newly released drug products.
16. *Physicians' Desk Reference*: Reference on pharmacology divided into seven sections. See p. 6 of textbook to further verify content of each section.
17. IV
18. IV
19. IV
20. II
21. II
22. II
23. III
24. III
25. III

26. II
27. II
28. The Controlled Substance Act of 1970 provides the legal basis for the drugs that are classified as controlled substances. This law establishes the degree of control, the conditions of recordkeeping, the particular order forms required, and other regulations relating to these drugs depending on classification.
29. Nurses must administer controlled substances under the direction of a physician or dentist who has been licensed to prescribe these agents. Nurses may not have a controlled substance in their possession unless 1) they have been requested to administer it to a patient under a doctor's order, 2) the nurse is the patient for whom the controlled substance was prescribed, or 3) the nurse is the official custodian of a limited supply of controlled substances on a patient care unit of a hospital.
30. *Tyler's Honest Herbal* contains monographs on 120 individual herbal names with information on the herb's use and the author's judgment with regard to rational clinical uses of the herb.
31. Answers will be individual, based on the clinical setting.

CHAPTER 2

1. F, parenteral
2. T

Copyright © 2001 by Mosby, Inc. All rights reserved.

3. T
4. T
5. F, percutaneous
6. T
7. F, do not stimulate a response.
8. T
9. F, inactivation of drug
10. T
11. T
12. F, metabolism
13. T
14. additive
15. synergistic
16. displacement
17. incompatibility
18. Drug tolerance occurs when increasingly larger doses are required to achieve the same effect that was achieved with a lesser dose previously.
19. Drug dependence means "addiction."
20. c
21. b
22. b
23. d
24. c
25. a

CHAPTER 3

1. T
2. F, not
3. F, does not have
4. T
5. F, does not
6. T
7. T
8. F, An elder has a lower percent of body fluid than an infant.
9. T
10. T
11. T
12. F, Bound drug is unable to cause a drug action.
13. F, Infants are babies 1–24 months of age.

CHAPTER 4

1. subjective
2. assessment
3. medication history
4. defining characteristics, actual nursing diagnosis
5. nursing actions/intervention

6. measurable goal statement
7. the exact time the last dose of the medication was administered
8. before
9. risk nursing diagnosis statements

CHAPTER 5

1. F, cognitive
2. T
3. T
4. T
5. F, not
6. T
7. F, referral may be necessary
8. T
9. T
10. T

CHAPTER 6 (PART 1)

1. 1
2. 3
3. 1
4. 2
5. 4
6. 1
7. 480
8. 60
9. 1
10. 1000
11. 1000
12. 1000
13. 15
14. multiply number of g by 15
15. divide number of gr by 15
16. divide by 1000; that is, move decimal point of milligrams three places to left
17. multiply the number of grains by 60 (60 mg/gr)

CHAPTER 6 (PART 2)

1. v
2. viiss
3. iv
4. xv
5. xx
6. xxiv
7. 1
8. 2
9. 3
10. 2
11. 10

12. 2 as written or 12 as improper fraction
13. 10
14. 3
15. 1/8
16. 3/4
17. 1/100
18. 1/3
19. 7/8
20. 1/90
21. 1/4
22. 1/2
23. 1/2
24. 3/4
25. 1 2/3
26. 3 2/5
27. 1 3/4
28. 12 3/4
29. 2 1/2
30. 1/3
31. 0.875= 0.88
32. 0.833= 0.83
33. 1.75
34. 0.666= 0.67
35. 0.9375= 0.94
36. 0.333= 0.33
37. 0.625= 0.63
38. 0.777= 0.78
39. 0.063= 0.06
40. 0.5
41. 1/12
42. 1/4
43. 7/16
44. 21/32
45. 2/7
46. 7/12
47. 1 1/8
48. 2 2/15
49. 0.76 = 0.8
50. 0.66 = 0.7
51. 2.22= 2.2
52. 17.70=17.7
53. 61.46= 61.5
54. 17.97=18
55. 1866.66= 1866.7
56. 3.81= 3.8
57. 33.83= 33.8
58. 0.56
59. 0.0066 = 0.66%
60. 66.6%
61. 0.75
62. 0.005
63. 75%
64. 87.5%
65. 1.23

Copyright © 2001 by Mosby, Inc.   All rights reserved.

66. 3/10
67. 3/1000
68. 3/100
69. 0.4
70. 0.04
71. 0.004
72. 3:4
73. 3:5
74. 1:200
75. 4
76. 16
77. 1
78. 30
79. 125
80. 360
81. 0.25
82. 4
83. 4 or 5
84. 2.73
85. 75

CHAPTER 7

1. d
2. a
3. e
4. c
5. ab
6. a
7. d
8. b
9. c
10. d
11. b
12. check school policy; usually false
13. c
14. d
15. c
16. b
17. a
18. b
19. d
20. d
21. See Figure 7-13, pp. 81
22. See textbook, pp. 82

CHAPTER 8

1. A capsule is a gelatin-type container holding dry or liquid drug.
2. Time-release tablets have layers of coating on the drug within the tablet so it dissolves at different rates.

3. oral; hold them in the mouth until they dissolve
4. water and alcohol
5. concentrated sugar with water
6. Emulsions are dispersed droplets throughout oil or water. Suspensions are liquid medications that require shaking before administration to disperse the insoluble drug throughout the solution.
7. 2
8. 5
9. F, Use accompanying dropper only; replace from pharmacy.
10. T
11. F, Clamp NG as fluid clears bottom of bulb syringe.
12. T
13. F, 24 hours
14. T
15. T
16. F, left
17. T
18. F, 1.0-6.0
19. F, yellow, bile-colored
20. F, Auscultation is not accurate.

CHAPTER 9

1. Figure 9-1
2. 0.5 ml
3. 1.4 ml
4. 2.2 ml
5. 1.7 ml
6. 52 U
7. 64 U
8. 11 U
9. 0.05 ml
10. 0.65 ml
11. 0.71 ml
12. 0.13 ml
13. Figure 9-8
14. 0.01-0.1
15. 0.5-2.0
16. 0.5-2.0; 2 to 3 ml (see note, Table 9-1)
17. 1000-2000 ml/24 hrs or as MD prescribes
18. 33
19. 31
20. 17
21. 31
22. Figure 9-15; textbook p. 106.
23. Figure 9-16, vial; textbook p. 106.
24. Figure 9-17, Mix-O-Vial; textbook p. 107.

25. Small piggyback bag higher than large primary bag; Figure 9-18, textbook p. 108.
26. Textbook
    a. intradermal 15° p. 116, Figure 9-25.
    b. subcutaneous 45° p. 118.
    c. intramuscular 90° p. 120, Figure 9-29.
27. Textbook, Figure 9-28; textbook p. 119.
28. Vastus lateralis; Figure 9-30; textbook p. 121.
29. Ventrogluteal; Figure 9-32; textbook p. 122.
30. IM injection sites; Figure 9-37; textbook p. 124.
31. Figures 9-33, 9-34, 9-35, textbook p. 123.
32. Use method and order of insulin withdrawal according to school or institution policy. See Figure 9-23; textbook pp. 114.
33. Back of hand, arms, dorsum of foot or the temporal region of the scalp; Figure 9-41; textbook p. 128.
34. SASH means saline flush, administer drug, saline flush, heparin flush; textbook p. 129.

CHAPTER 10

1. See textbook p. 140.
2. See textbook p. 140.
3. lotions
4. See textbook p. 140. Charting should be checked with the instructor of the course.
5. See textbook p. 143. Charting checked by instructor.
6. See textbook p. 143-144.
7. Have M.T. put the call light on whenever using the nitroglycerin. Obtain data regarding location, degree of pain being experienced and relief obtained. As appropriate, take and record vital signs. Chart symptoms present, degree of relief, number of nitroglycerin tablets used for each attack, and vital signs.
8. See charting—checked by instructor.
9. See textbook pp. 147-149.

Copyright © 2001 by Mosby, Inc. All rights reserved.

10. If inner canthus is not blocked, eye drops would drain immediately from eye without coming in contact with the eye surface and being absorbed.
11. In a child under three years, the earlobe is pulled downward and back; in an adult, it is pulled upward and back.
12. Gently blowing the nose clears nasal passages and allows better contact and absorption of medication via mucous membrane.
13. Overuse of some nasal sprays causes "rebound" effect that will cause worsening of symptoms. If drug is not effective, call pharmacist or physician; do not increase the number of drops or frequency of taking the medication.
14. See textbook pp. 152-153.
15. See textbook pp. 153-155.

CHAPTER 11

1. norepinephrine, epinephrine, dopamine
2. kidneys, brain, and gastrointestinal tract
3. alpha, beta, and dopaminergic
4. parasympathetic
5. smooth muscle relaxation; bronchodilation
6. smooth muscle contraction; bronchoconstriction
7. vitals; blood pressure, check for use of bronchodilators and decongestants
8. tachycardia, orthostatic hypotension, dizziness, tremors, flushed skin
9. dryness of mucous membranes, urinary retention, constipation
10. "olol"
11. See textbook, p. 165.
12. See textbook, p. 162.
13. See textbook, p. 162.
14. See textbook, p. 163.

Chapter 11 Math Review

1. 16 ml
2. 1 1/2 tablets
3. 0.4 mg; l ml

CHAPTER 12

1. initial insomnia
2. terminal insomnia
3. hypnotic
4. sedative
5. intermittent
6. hypnotic
7. Nursing Diagnosis: Sleep pattern disturbance r/t insufficient data m/b inability to sleep through the night
8. Nursing Diagnosis: Knowledge deficit related to hypnotic action/therapy m/b lack of understanding of long-term use of hypnotics for nightly sleep disturbances
9. Barbiturates: hangover, sedation, lethargy
   Benzodiazepines: drowsiness, hangover, sedation, lethargy
10. Physical dependence to a drug is when the individual cannot function effectively without the drug.
11. See Review Sheet, Sedative/Hypnotics, pp. 66-67 of the Student Learning Guide.

Chapter 12 Math Review

1. 2 tablets of 0.25 mg. General rule, when two dosages are available, give the least number of tablets which accurately fills the prescribed amount.
2. 4 ml of 500 mg/5ml syrup or 8 ml of 250 mg/5 ml chloral hydrate. Neither of capsules, 250 mg or 500 mg, can be given to accurately prepare the ordered dose.
3. Safe dosage range is between 6 mg and 9 mg, therefore prescribed amount of 7.5 mg is reasonable.

CHAPTER 13

1. dopamine; acetylcholine
2. regain dopaminergic activity as close to normal level of functioning; reduce symptoms of disease, thereby increasing the individual's quality of life
3. See textbook, p. 178.

4. Variable responses possible; check with instructor.
5. monitoring blood pressure q shift; provide for patient safety, etc.
6. Assess orientation to name, place, date, time and basic functioning; e.g., confusion, alertness, etc.
7. Response time may vary and dosage will be individualized; response may not be immediate.
8. anticholinergic
9. See textbook, p. 175.
10. to reduce metabolism of levodopa
11. to cross into brain and be metabolized to dopamine to help restore deficient dopamine levels
12. reduces destruction of dopamine in peripheral tissue making more dopamine available in the brain

Chapter 13 Math Review

1. one tablet per dose of 25/100 strength
2. 1 tablet, 250 mg per dose of 250 mg strength
3. 1/2 tablet of 2.5 mg strength per dose

CHAPTER 14

1-6. See textbook, pp. 192-193.
7. See textbook, pp. 193-194.
8. Provide for patient safety while intervening to reduce panic level.
9. Benzodiazepines
   Action: Stimulates neurotransmitter GABA that will reduce anxiety level
   Side effects: CNS depression (e.g., drowsiness, sedation, lethargy)
10. Azaspirones
   Action: Midbrain modulator whose action is not fully understood; it is a partial serotonin agonist
   Side effects: CNS depression (e.g., drowsiness, sedation, lethargy)

Copyright © 2001 by Mosby, Inc.   All rights reserved.

11. Hydroxyzine
Action: Antihistamine with several actions on CNS (See textbook, p. 189)
Side effects: CNS depression (e.g., sedation) and anticholinergic activity (e.g., blurred vision, dryness of mucosa, constipation, urinary hesitancy)
12. Meprobamate
Action: Unknown mechanism of action
Side effects: CNS depression (e.g., sedation, lethargy, drowsiness)
Note that all of these drugs act on the CNS to produce some degree of depression.
13. Level of anxiety present, vital signs, including blood pressure in sitting and supine positions; check for a history of blood dyscrasias or hepatic disease; determine if the patient is in the first trimester of pregnancy or breast-feeding.

Chapter 14 Math Review

1. 0.8 ml
2. 400 mg/dose
3. 0.75 ml

CHAPTER 15

1. euphoria or elation
2. depression
3. MAOIs
4. SSRIs
5. tricyclic antidepressants
6. miscellaneous agents (e.g., bupropion hydrochloride)
7. blood pressure and pulse
8. baseline blood sugar (diabetics)
9. meals with tyramine content
10. medical history (e.g., levodopa)
11. extrapyramidal symptoms
12. to check for therapeutic response
13. blocking reuptake or destruction of neurotransmitters (norepinephrine, dopamine, serotonin)
14. tyramine
15. SSRIs

16. the drug's anticholinergic effects (e.g., blurred vision, constipation, urinary retention, dry mucosa)
17. sedation
18. orthostatic hypotension
19. lab tests (e.g., electrolytes, FBS, BUN, creatinine clearance, urinalysis, thyroid function)
20. blood pressure
21. baseline weight and hydration status
22. signs of sodium depletion
23. 0.4 to 1.5 mEq/L.

Chapter 15 Math Review

1. 2 tablets
2. Dosage available: 25, 50, 75 mg tablets. Most likely 50 mg dispensed for this order. The 100 mg dose would require 2 tablets (50 mg strength)

CHAPTER 16

1. d
2. ab
3. a
4. c
5. e
6. See textbook p. 219.
7. See textbook p. 221, and instructor.
8. See textbook p. 220; site, degree of sedation, EPS, hypotension, and anticholinergic effects.
9. Neutropenia present. Report sore throat, jaundice, progressive weakness.
10. to prevent EPS
11. sedation, orthostatic hypotension, anticholinergic effects
12. site/instructor specific
13. Thorazine
14. perphenazine
15. thioridazine
16. Clozaril
17. haloperidol

Chapter 16 Math Review

1. 6.3 ml
2. 2 tabs
3. 0.6 ml of 20 mg/ml or 1.2 ml of 10 mg/ml

CHAPTER 17

1. barbiturates, benzodiazepines, hydantoins, succinimides
2. increases seizure threshold and regulates neuronal firing in brain
3. tonic phase—loss of consciousness, body rigidity, intense muscle contractions clonic phase—alternate jerking and relaxation of extremities
4. benzodiazepines
5. hyperglycemia
6. Phenytoin, Tegretol, Primidone
7. antacid
8. See textbook, pp. 229-230.
9. hypotension, dyspnea, edema, neurologic nephrotoxicity, hepatotoxicity, blood dyscrasias, dermatologic reactions

Chapter 17 Math Review

1. Need to clarify order. What is the route of administration? What form of drug is to be used? Available in 50 mg tablets; 30 and 100 mg capsules; suspension 30 and 125 mg/5 ml; and in 50 mg/ml injectable form. Give 100 mg Dilantin capsules three times per day and at hs if po route is used,
Schedule: 8:00 A.M., 1:00 P.M., 6:00 PM, 10:00 P.M. (hs)
2. Using an oral syringe, measure 2.5 ml of Tegretol suspension to administer 50 mg. Give po approximately every 6 hours.
3. Yes, this is a reasonable order. Depakene is only available in oral form. At 15 mg/kg/24 hr, and 110 lb (50 kg), this means a total daily dose of 750 mg/24 hr or 250 mg, tid. Depakene syrup is available as 250 mg/5 ml. Give 5 ml, three times per day at 7:00 A.M., 2:00 P.M., and 10:00 P.M. (The later dose would maintain more consistent blood level.)

CHAPTER 18

1. awareness of the sensation of pain

Copyright © 2001 by Mosby, Inc.   All rights reserved.

2. level at which pain is first felt
3. drugs that relieve pain without producing loss of consciousness
4. See textbook, pp. 242-243.
5. baseline neurologic assessment: vital signs, voiding and bowel pattern, prior use of analgesics, pain assessment
6. no
7. sedation, light-headedness, nausea and vomiting, sweating, orthostatic hypotension, constipation
8. for reversal of CNS depression effects of opiate agonists, opiate partial agonists and propoxyphene
9. gastric irritation
10. No, it is not an anti-inflammatory agent.
11. 21
12. 83
13. when the patient has abnormal liver function, or the drug causes these effects
14. salicylism; tinnitus, impaired hearing, decreased vision, sweating, fever, lethargy, dizziness, mental confusion, nausea and vomiting
15. nalmefene, naloxone, naltrexone

Chapter 18 Math Review

1. 2 tablets
2. 3.8 ml
3. Give 1 ml, 15 mg/ml morphine
4. Does not say po; clarify order. Also, is this drug required qid or better on a q4h prn basis?

CHAPTER 19

1. fluvastatin, lovastatin, pravastatin, simvastatin, atorvastatin, cervistatin
2. decreased LDL, decreased total cholesterol, decreased triglycerides, increased HDLs
3. may cause hyperglycemia
4. baseline cholesterol, triglycerides, FBS (gemfibrozil), any GI symptoms present, and liver function studies
5. fat-soluble vitamins (DEAK)
6. Digitalis: bradycardia and control of heart disorder would

decline. Warfarin: anticoagulant properties would decline and the patient would be prone to signs and symptoms of clot formation.

Chapter 19 Math Review

1. Give 1 tablet/dose (500 mg tablet)
   Total: 1500 mg daily
2. 4 tablets

CHAPTER 20

1. pulse pressure
2. peripheral resistance
3. vasoconstriction; increased peripheral resistance
4. thiazide and thiazide-like diuretics, loop diuretics
5. monitor for hypoglycemia; symptoms may be blocked by actions of beta-adrenergic agents
6. hypotension, dizziness, tachycardia, fainting
7. ACE Inhibitors
8. Since these drugs act on renin-angiotensin system they can cause fetal and neonatal harm especially during the second and third trimester of pregnancy.
9. Calcium ion antagonists relax smooth muscles of blood vessels resulting in lowering of blood pressure.
10. ACE Inhibitors
11. angiotensin II receptor antagonists
12. See textbook, pp. 276-277.
13. See textbook, pp. 276-277.
14. Infuse 60 gtt/min

Chapter 20 Math Review

1. Call pharmacy and ask that 0.3 mg tablets be provided. Would only need 2 tabs of 0.3 mg Otherwise, 3 tablets of 0.2 mg strength or 6 tablets of 0.1 mg tablets could be administered. If ordering the 0.3 mg strength, explain to the patient that they will receive a different number of tablets when the new strength is on the unit.
2. 2 tabs dose
   9:00 A.M. and 9:00 P.M. or 0900 and 2100

CHAPTER 21

1. negative chronotropy
2. positive chronotropy
3. digitalization
4. apical; one full
5. after meals; gastric irritation
6. Improves circulation and cardiac output by slowing and strengthening force of each condition.
7. See textbook, pp. 298, 300.
8. See Chapter 20.

Chapter 21 Math Review

1. 75 kg
   450 mcg or 0.45 mg
   Digoxin may be administered undiluted; or each 1 ml may be diluted in 4 ml sterile water. IV dose should be given slowly over at least five minutes. Give with caution with hypertension because IV administration may elevate the blood pressure. It is compatible with normal saline, 5% D/W, or lactated Ringer's solution.
2. Give 0.5 ml of 0.25 mg/ml
3. Two alternatives:
   -Give 1 tablet of 0.25 mg and 1 tablet of 0.125 mg or
   -Give 3 tablets of 0.125 mg digoxin
   Which method would be the most accurate? Discuss with the clinical instructor.

CHAPTER 22

1. restore normal sinus rhythm
2. restore normal cardiac functioning
3. prevent life-threatening arrhythmias
4. poor tissue perfusion to brain cells
5. depresses myocardium by preventing sodium ion movement
6. Prolongs duration of electrical stimulation on cells and the refractory time between electrical impulses.
7. decreases heart rate

Copyright © 2001 by Mosby, Inc.   All rights reserved.

8. decreases systolic blood pressure
9. decreases cardiac output
10. Local anesthetic lidocaine contains a preservative and some have epinephrine added; either of which may be harmful to a patient with an arrhythmia.
11. rash, chills, fever, tinnitus from quinidine
12. SA node to AV node to Bundle of His to Purkinje fibers to the heart tissue of the myocardium
13. electrocardiogram
14. dyspnea
15. fatigue
16. edema
17. chest pain
18. syncope
19. palpitations

Chapter 22 Math Review

1. 4 tablets/dose
   2.4 g in 24 hours
2. 4 capsules/dose

CHAPTER 23

1. See textbook, p. 316.
2. See textbook, p. 317.
3. See textbook, p. 318.
4. Up to 3 tablets in 15 minute period (5 minutes apart) sublingual. If no relief seek additional treatment from physician or an emergency room.
5. q 8-12 h
6. One tablet tid, one on arising, pc lunch and pc evening meal.
7. See textbook, pp. 319-321; and Chapter 10, Percutaneous Administration.
8. See review sheet question 6.
9. See Table 23-2 and Table 11-3.
10. See textbook, pp. 319, 322.

Chapter 23 Math Review

1. 2 tablets
2. 1 capsule
   Sublingual administration; puncture capsule with needle and squeeze medication under tongue.
3. 2 ml

CHAPTER 24

1. See textbook, pp. 327-328.
2. See textbook, pp. 326-327.
3. See textbook, pp. 325-326.
4. Improved tissue perfusion, decreased pain, increased exercise tolerance, and improved peripheral pulses.

Chapter 24 Math Review

1. 200 mg dose x 4 days requires 16 tablets 400 mg dose x next 5 days requires 10 tablets
2. 2 capsules per dose

CHAPTER 25

1. Heart failure
2. Hypertension
3. Hematocrit
4. Hemoglobin
5. BUN
6. Electrolytes (also skin turgor, I/O, breath sounds, others)
7. 135-145 mEq/liter
8. 3.5-4.7 mEq/liter
9. Furosemide
10. Loop diuretics
11. Hyperglycemia
12. Hyperuricemia
13. Orthostatic hypotension or dehydration
14.-16. Bumetanide Bumex), ethacrynic acid (Edecrin), furosemide (Lasix) or torsemide (Demadex)
17.-19. See Table 25-1, 25-2
20. Amiloride (Midamor), spironolactone (Aldactone), or triamterene (Dyrenium)
21. Data to be used as a baseline for comparison with subsequent data to evaluate response to diuretic therapy.
22. Increased uric acid secretion may result in hyperuricemia; prevented by administering allopurinol especially in patients who have a history of previous gouty arthritis attacks.
23. Potassium and sodium; occasionally magnesium
24. Diuretics can cause excessive excretion of potassium resulting in hypokalemia and loss of fluid

can cause increased concentration of the digoxin in the fluids leading to digitalis toxicity.
25. Aminoglycosides
26. Furosemide and torsemide = loop diuretics
   Hydrochlorothiazide = thiazide diuretic
   Spironolactone = potassium-sparing diuretic
27. Combination diuretics contain both a thiazide and potassium sparing diuretic in an attempt to prevent hypokalemia associated with the use of a thiazide-like diuretic alone.

Chapter 25 Math Review

1. 100 ml/hr
2. 2 tablets

CHAPTER 26

1. Embolus
2. Thrombus
3. Platelet inhibitors and anticoagulants
4. Fibrinolytic agents
5. APTT
6. 1.5 to 2.5 times the control APTT value.
7. Daily platelet counts
8. Periodic CBC
9. Stools for occult blood
10. Bleeding at any site
11. Signs and symptoms of shock
12. Blood in stools or urine
13. Platelet count at or below 100,000 mm^3
14. Vitamin K
15. b
16. c
17. 8 ml/hr
18. 80 gtts/min

Chapter 26 Math Review

1. 0.2 ml
2. 2.7 ml/hr
   2400 U have already infused.
   4 ml/hr
3. 28 tablets

CHAPTER 27

1. Vasoconstriction

Copyright © 2001 by Mosby, Inc. All rights reserved.

2. Following prescribed dosage and duration of therapy
3. Antihistamines or H₂ receptor antagonists
4. On a regular schedule whether an allergen is present; antigen
5. Textbook, p. 366.
6. See Chapter 10, pp. 150-153.

CHAPTER 28

1. Textbook, p. 369.
2. Textbook, p. 369.
3. Textbook, p. 372.
4. Textbook, p. 372.
5. Liquefy mucus
6. Suppress cough center in brain
7. Acts directly on mucus plug(s) to reduce thickness and/or dissolve mucus plug(s).
8. Textbook, pp. 373-374.
9. Textbook, p. 385.
10. Textbook, pp. 382, 384.
11. Figure 28-3, pp. 374-375.
12. Textbook, p. 388.

Chapter 28 Math Review

1. 9.4 ml or 2.7 tsp using equivalent of 4 ml/tsp or 1.8 tsp using equivalent 5 ml/tsp.
2. 0.25 ml.
3. Give 87.95 = 88 mg/*individual dose.*
4. Give 8.8 ml/*individual dose.*

CHAPTER 29

1. Cold sores caused by herpes simplex type 1 virus.
2. Fungal infection caused by *Candida albicans.*
3. Foul odor from the mouth.
4. Partial or complete stoppage of saliva in mouth.
5.-9. Lidocaine
   Milk of Magnesia
   Kaopectate
   Nystatin liquid or clotrimazole
   Lozenges
   Sucralfate suspension
   Oral or parenteral analgesics

CHAPTER 30

1. F, ineffective
2. T
3. F, increases pH
4. T
5. T
6. T
7. F, coats ulcer crater
8. F, increases peristalsis
9. T
10. See Table 30-3, p. 409.
11. See Table 30-2, p. 403.
12. 2.5 ml
13. 1 tab ac
    2 tabs at hs

Chapter 30 Math Review

1. 300 ml/hr
2. 0.875 = 0.88 ml

CHAPTER 31

1. A pregnant woman with persistent vomiting that affects electrolyte fluid and nutritional status
2. Self-induced vomiting or in response to an unpleasant stimulus
3. Chemotherapy-induced emesis
4. Suppression of vomiting center
5. Interruption of impulses going to or from vomiting center
6. Inhibits dopamine receptors in pathway to vomiting center
7. CIE and postoperative nausea and vomiting
8. Motion sickness
9. As soon as nausea is initially experienced
10. Stimulation of labyrinth system of the ear with subsequent transmission of stimulus to vomiting center
11. 24 to 120 hours
12. Dopamine antagonists, serotonin antagonists, anticholinergic agents, corticosteroids, benzodiazepines, cannabinoids
13. See textbook, p. 413.
14. See textbook, p. 415—dopamine antagonists
    See textbook, p. 415—serotonin antagonists

See textbook, p. 420—anticholinergic agents
See textbook, p. 420—corticosteroids
See textbook, p. 421—benzodiazepines
See textbook, p. 421—cannabinoids

Chapter 31 Math Review

1. 61.36 kg; 9.2 mg of ondansetron; set infusion pump to 150 ml/hr.
2. 1.5 ml

CHAPTER 32

1. Retains H₂O in stool, stimulates peristalsis
2. Softens stool and lubricates intestinal mucosa, peristalsis not increased
3. Adsorbs excess H₂O to cause stool to be formed
4. Decreased peristalsis and GI motility
5. Foods contaminated with bacteria or protozoa or contaminated drinking water.
6. High-fiber diet with adequate fluids for hydration, especially water
7. Magnesium
8. Bulk-forming laxatives

CHAPTER 33

1. F, does
2. T
3. F, hyperglycemic
4. T
5. F, 50-60% CHO
   30% fats
   10-20% proteins
6. F, hypoglycemia
7. T
8. F, too little food intake
9. F, may require insulin during stress, illness, infections
10. T
11. F, 8-10 week period
12. F, Hyperglycemia may require hospitalization with stabilization of electrolytes, fluid balance and insulin levels via IV

Copyright © 2001 by Mosby, Inc. All rights reserved.

administration, not subcutaneous administration of insulin.
13. F, blocks symptoms of hypoglycemia
14. T
15. T
16. 2-4 ounces fruit juice with 2 tsp sugar or honey, 1 cup of skim milk, 4 ounces nondiet soft drink, or 1 piece of candy (not chocolate)
17. insulin
monitoring of blood glucose and ketones
hospitalization
identify underlying cause
If severe, usually requires rehydration and normalization of electrolytes.
18. the brain
19. regular
20. ultralente
21. refrigerated except current bottle in use at room temperature
22. cannot; Regular insulin is the only insulin approved for IV administration at this time.

Chapter 33 Math Review

1. Volume of NPH:
0.22 ml. Can use TB syringe or measure 22 U NPH in a U-100 insulin syringe
2. a. Volume of NPH:
0.27 ml. Use TB syringe or 27 units NPH in a U-100 insulin syringe
   b. Volume of regular insulin:
0.07 ml. Use TB syringe or 7 U in a U-100 insulin syringe
   c. Total volume to inject:
0.27 ml NPH plus 0.07 ml regular = 0.34 ml or a total of 34 U (27 NPH + 7 U regular)

CHAPTER 34

1. T
2. F, Replaces T_3, T_4 hormones that are deficient.
3. T
4. F, hypoactive
5. F, high

6. F, weight gain
7. See textbook pp. 451-453.

Chapter 34 Math Review

1. 2 tablets
2. 0.2 mg

CHAPTER 35

1. F, Adrenal cortex
2. T
3. T
4. T
5. F, Does mask signs and symptoms of infection.
6. T
7. T
8. F, 6 AM–9 AM
9. T

Chapter 35 Math Review

1. 10 Kg
2. 1 mg; 1.5 mg

CHAPTER 36

1. Testes
2. Ovaries
3. Fostering implantation
4. Fertilization of ovum and maintaining pregnancy
5. Preparing breast for lactation
6. Pregnant or not
7. Weight
8. Vital signs, especially blood pressure
9. History of thromboembolic disorders or cancer of reproductive organs
10. Maturation of ovarian follicle
11. Inhibit ovulation
12. Masculinization

Chapter 36 Math Review

1. 1.5 ml
2. 0.2 ml

CHAPTER 37

1. See textbook pp. 489-490.
2. See textbook p. 490.
3. See textbook p. 475.
4. See textbook p. 489.
5. 10% calcium gluconate
6. See textbook p. 491.

7. See textbook p. 491.
8. See textbook p. 485.

Chapter 37 Math Review

1. Available 0.2 mg/ml
Give 1 ml
2. 62.5 ml/hr

CHAPTER 38

1. Estrogen and progestin
2. 21 days
3. Every day
4. Minipill
5-9. Nausea, headache, weight gain, spotting, depression, fatigue, chloasma, yeast infections, vaginal itching or discharge, alterations in libido
10. See textbook, p. 496. Patient Education and Health Promotion.
11. Phenobarbital, ampicillin, isoniazid, rifampin, benzodiazepines, primidone, and carbamazepine
12. Alpha$_1$ adrenergic blocking agents and antiandrogen agents
13. Obtain a baseline PSA blood level before finasteride therapy. This drug decreases the PSA level by about 50% in patients with BPH, even in the presence of prostatic cancer.
14. Assess vital signs and check for cardiovascular disease history. Do not administer without checking with a physician if the vital signs are abnormal or there is a history of cardiovascular disease.

Chapter 38 Math Review

1. 1000 mg; 70 capsules
2. 11 capsules

CHAPTER 39

1. See textbook, pp. 508-509.
2. Reddish-orange
3. Administering Vitamin C
4. Quinolone antibiotics
5. Formaldehyde
6. False
7. Rust-brown to yellow
8. Nonobstructive urine retention

Copyright © 2001 by Mosby, Inc. All rights reserved.

9. Fosfomycin (Monurol)
10. Acidic
11. Vitamin C
12. Tinted rust-brown to yellow
13. Urecholine or bethanechol chloride

Chapter 39 Math Review

1. 0.5 ml
2. 7.5 ml

CHAPTER 40

1. os
2. od
3. ou
4. Block inner canthus
5. 1 to 2
6. Acetylcholine
7. Miosis
8. Dilation (mydriasis)
9. Reduce volume of intraocular fluid
10. Decrease production of aqueous humor
11. Hazy vision, lacrimation, redness and burning of eyes, and sensitivity to bright lights
12. Allergic reaction of the eye and other acute, noninfectious inflammatory conditions
13. Carbonic anhydrase inhibitors inhibit the enzyme carbonic anhydrase, which results in a decrease of aqueous humor production thereby lowering IOP.
14. Patients with a respiratory condition (e.g., bronchitis, emphysema, asthma) because beta blockers may produce severe bronchoconstriction. Use in patients with heart failure should be limited to those persons whose disease is under control because hypotension, bradycardia, and/or heart failure may develop with use of these agents.

Chapter 40 Math Review

1. 156 lbs. equals 70.9 kg
   Total dose is: 106 g.

CHAPTER 41

1. Discuss with instructor.
2. Post sign on patient door: "neutropenic precautions," initiate nursing interventions, and update the plan of care. See textbook, pp. 508
3. Nonspecific
4. Specific, s phase
5. Specific, during mitosis
6. Eradication of malignant cells
7. See textbook chapter 31.
8. Skin turgor (not an accurate indicator in the elderly), mucous membrane moistness, softness vs. firmness of eyeballs, electrolyte reports, fluid balance (I & O)
9. See textbook, p. 545.
10. 80 gtts/min
11. 61.4 kg
12. 307 mcg
13. 1.02 ml = 1 ml
14. Ifosfamide and cyclophosphamide, bladder tissue
15. Platelets
16. Breast cancer with HER2-positive tumors

Chapter 41 Math Review

1. 100 ml/per hour
2. Check directions on type of PCA pump used in the clinical setting where you are assigned and discuss method of initiating PCA pump setting and of recording amount of morphine sulfate used in narcotics records.

CHAPTER 42

1. Check vital signs, respiratory assessment, swallowing, gag reflex.
2. Check with anesthesiologist before giving analgesic.
3. Check with instructor.
4. Immobilization, elevation of injured body part as appropriate to location of injury, application of ice pack
5. Used in combination with physical therapy, rest, and analgesics to relieve muscle spasms associated with acute, painful musculoskeletal conditions
6. Vital signs, mental status data, lab studies (e.g., CBC, liver function studies as ordered by physician)
7. Vital signs, especially temperature and extent of muscle symptoms present

Chapter 42 Math Review

1. 1500 mg

CHAPTER 43

1. To prevent development of resistant organisms
2. Rifampin (Rifadin)
3. Gm+ and Gm-
4. Prior allergies to medications, food, or asthma; obtain details of the signs and symptoms that developed during the allergic reaction
5. Inhibit protein synthesis of bacterial cell wall
6. Interfere with synthesis of bacterial cell wall
7. During last half of pregnancy or while breastfeeding; do not administer to children until permanent teeth are in place (usually by age 8 years)
8. Inhibit bacterial protein synthesis
9. Sulfonamides
10. Kaopectate; physician should be consulted.
11. See textbook, p. 581.
12. See textbook, p. 579.
13. See textbook, pp. 584-585.
14. Rifampin
15. Streptogramins
16. These organisms grow in the absence of oxygen.
17. ototoxicity and nephrotoxicity
18. Perform baseline assessment of presenting symptoms, allergies, T, P, R, BP, and state of hydration. Check laboratory studies available that relate to the client's condition or disease process. Check individual drug monographs for specific

Copyright © 2001 by Mosby, Inc.   All rights reserved.

assessments as they relate to the prescribed antibiotic.

19. Patients allergic to sulfa may also have a cross-sensitivity to sulfonylurea oral hypoglycemic agents.

20. Weaken the microorganism, allowing the patient's individual immune system to finish combating the infection

21. During last half of pregnancy and for children through eight years of age, tetracycline may permanently stain the teeth. (It is also excreted in breast milk, so do not administer to a nursing mother.)

22. See textbook, pp. 582, 584-585.

23. Oral administration is every 4 hours around the clock.

Chapter 43 Math Review

1. Infant weight is 5.9 kg.
   295 mg.
   Each divided dose is 73.7 mg = 74 mg.
   Give 0.74 ml, using a tuberculin syringe

2. Give: 6 ml.
3. Give: 1.2 ml.
4. 25 gtts/minute
5. 100 ml/hr

CHAPTER 44

1. F, do *not* meet needs of ill patients
2. F, calculate basal energy expenditure in kcal per day
3. F, 3-5.5 g/kg/day
4. T
5. T
6. T
7. T
8. T
9. F, Osmolyte is used for tube feedings.
10. T
11. T
12. F, every 8 hours or by institutional policy
13. T
14. T
15. T
16. T
17. T

18. F, PPN
19. F, require central line or port
20. F, neuropathy
21. T
22. F, should not be used
23. T

Chapter 44 Math Review

1. Increase hourly rate by 11.4 ml/hr to a total of 91.4 or 91 ml. hour
2. 2400 ml

CHAPTER 45

1. See textbook, p. 613.
2. See textbook, p. 613.
3. Instructor-student-classroom discussion
4. Open textbook activity
5. Antihypertensives and hormone replacement products
6. Nonspecific immune
7. Reducing high blood pressure, hypercholesterolemia; also affects platelet aggregation
8. Saw palmetto

Copyright © 2001 by Mosby, Inc.   All rights reserved.